Determined, Dedicated, Disciplined
To Be Fit

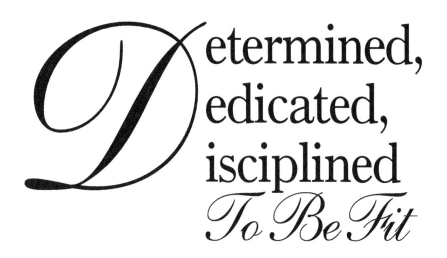

Determined, Dedicated, Disciplined To Be Fit

The "Ageless" Journey of Ernestine Shepherd

ERNESTINE SHEPHERD

Written with Theresa Royal Brown

ISBN-10: 0-9978541-0-3

ISBN-13: 978-0-9978541-0-7

All Scripture quotations are taken from the King James Version of the Bible.

Book Ghostwritten, Published, Coordinated and Arranged by:
Theresa Royal Brown
Royal Brown Publishing

Recent Pictures Throughout Book of Ernestine Shepherd Taken By:
Marvin Joseph

Work Out Chapter Pictures and Older Picture Scans Done By:
Maynard Manzano
Magic Glamor Photography

Exercise and Nutrition Input By:
Yohnnie Shambourger
Yohnnex Sports, Inc.

SPECIAL NOTE: To all corporations, universities, colleges and professional organizations: Quantity discounts are available on bulk purchases of this book for educational, gift purposes or as premiums for increasing magazine subscriptions or renewals. Email info@agelessjourneybook.com for bulk order information.

$\mathcal{P}$raise for Determined, Dedicated, Disciplined To Be Fit– The Ageless Journey of Ernestine Shepherd:

"I read your book in 2 days. I honestly felt like we were having a conversation and you were telling me your story. I am 57 years old and need to get Determined, Dedicated, and Disciplined To Be Fit! I'm so sorry about your sister Dim's passing but love that you kept her by your side all these years. I hope to see and meet you on your book tour. It really is a wonderful book. Thank you and God bless you." (R. Galvan)

"I am 58 years young and just finished reading "Determined, Dedicated, Disciplined To Be Fit". This book has deeply touched me and is an inspiration to me now as I am getting started on my own fitness journey and will continue to be as I travel down this road. My sister, Mary, and I started training for a 5K two months ago and will be running it next Saturday. I also signed up with a local gym and have a renewed determination to make lifelong changes regarding all things about fitness. Thanks to everyone who helped her help others. What a story, what a life, what a gift and a blessing. I am forever grateful!" (J. Owen)

"I love the book Ms.Ernestine! I cannot put it down. We need a movie! I will pray that it will come to pass. Your story is something that our children will be inspired by. God Bless You! Love you!" (J. Winbush)

"On Friday, I received your book in the mail. Today is Saturday and I finished reading every page. You are a remarkable woman. I laughed, cried & journeyed along with you as I read each chapter of your life. Blessings to you & all those who helped you share your story." (C. McMichael)

"Just got your book and can not put it down!!! Thank you!" (B. Bradley)

"I received my signed copy. Feeling so blessed. The struggles and sentiments resonate deeply with me. I'm am humbled and ashamed that I've not been doing the three D's to date, but on reading through your journey so far, I have renewed intent. Truly a great inspirational lady. Thank you!" (P. Andrews)

"Can't put it down! She's the real live Rocky!" (B. Gannon)

"I am reading your book, and it feels like you are right here with me telling your story. You are such a blessing." (K. Hartsfield)

"Received your book yesterday, and I finished it today. I couldn't put it down, it was so inspiring. I'm almost 59 and have been working out in the gym for 4 years. I've been through back issues, hip issues, knee issues but keep pushing. I used to walk a lot like you, but due to a hip issue, I can no longer walk very far. I have now taken up bicycling and enjoy it more than walking. I really enjoyed reading your book and it has made me realize, I can lose the weight, I just need to be determined, dedicated and disciplined and make it my life. Thank you again for the inspiration." (K. Sutherlin)

Dedication

This book is dedicated to my wonderful husband Shep and my son Michael. I thank you for all the love and support you have given me throughout the years. You are the wind beneath my wings and I love you both very much.

Teeny

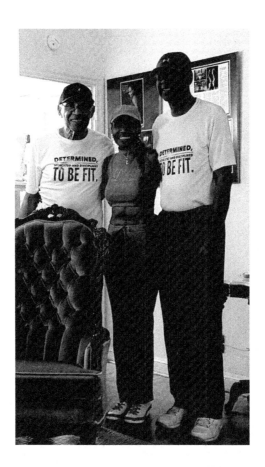

Table of Contents

1
Introduction

3
Chapter 1
The Hawkins Family and the Rise of Little Ernestine

25
Chapter 2
Shep and Michael … The Two Loves of My Life

43
Chapter 3
The Journey Into Fitness

$\mathcal{I}$ntroduction

As I STOOD THERE BEHIND THE CURTAIN, ready to go out to do my 5th body building competition, I couldn't help but think, "How did I get here, and how has God shown so much favor to a little girl from Baltimore?"

As with my first competition, a little bit of fear gripped me and a lot of questions came to my mind. "Will they like me? Am I good enough? Do I deserve to be here?" I closed my eyes, just as I had done with all the competitions in the past, took a deep breath and breathed through the fear. I then straightened my back, smiled one of my biggest smiles and walked out on that stage.

Who am I? How did a 56 year old woman start a body building journey that has spanned over a 24-year period? How have I gotten to this place and still continue even as I near 80 years young?

Are you ready to go on a journey with me? Are you ready to find out how I became Determined, Dedicated and Disciplined to be fit for life? Do you want to know how you can do it too?

It hasn't been a straight road, and there have been some twists and turns along the way; however, I know I have truly been blessed. My story is still being written, but if you are ready to go on this journey with me, I am ready to share.

Are you ready?

Ok, here we go...

$\mathcal{C}$hapter 1
The Hawkins Family and the Rise of Little Ernestine

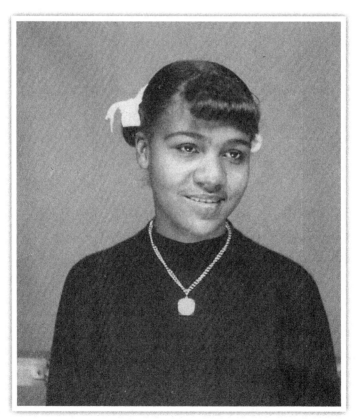

My picture at age 15.
Photo credit: Ernestine Shepherd

Ernestine Blondine Hawkins (Shepherd)

EVERY JOURNEY HAS A BEGINNING AND GOD ordained
mine to start on June 16, 1936. I was born in Baltimore,
MD to two wonderful parents, Milton Augustus Hawkins
and Ernestine Blondine Hawkins, who I was named after.
Everyone said I was cute, but from looking at some of my
younger pictures, I have to say no way! I looked "ok" but
never really had the best self-esteem as a child. I was very
nervous and would bite my finger nails until they bled
and I also bit my toenails, yes my toenails! I had no confidence and I lived in a make-believe world. For some reason,
I always needed to be reassured that my parents loved me
to the point that I think it was overwhelming for them. I
needed that attention and reassurance CONSTANTLY, and
it was a bit too much. Now that I am older, I often reflect
back on that time in my life, and wonder why I felt that
I never quite "fit in". I think sometimes "middle" children
may feel this way more than the oldest child or the youngest
child because being in the middle, well, you are just in the
middle. I now understand that my constant craving for love
and attention was simply feelings of low self-esteem. Have
any of you ever felt like that growing up? Like you didn't fit
in, like no one really understood you, like you just needed to
be reassured over and over that you did matter and that you
were loved. Low self-esteem makes you do things and feel

things that those with high self-esteem would never dream of doing or feeling. I still struggle with where the origin of those feelings of low self-esteem came from, but I am thankful I have "outgrown" them.

There were 6 children in total and we all had the same parents. My brothers and sisters from the oldest to the youngest are as follows: Eleanora (Dee), Mildred (Dim/Velvet) – (Deceased), Ernestine (Teeny/Tootsie), Milton (Mick), Robert (Bobby) – (Deceased) and Bernice (Bunny). I loved and still love each of them very much.

My father started out working at a box factory but ended up being a small business owner. In those days we didn't have much money but my parents made sure we had everything we needed, and we made it. Dad was a very fair skin person but for his body he was small but had great biceps and back muscles. He was also a very kind man and everyone that met my dad really loved him. I always try very hard to be kind to people and I know I definitely got that from my daddy.

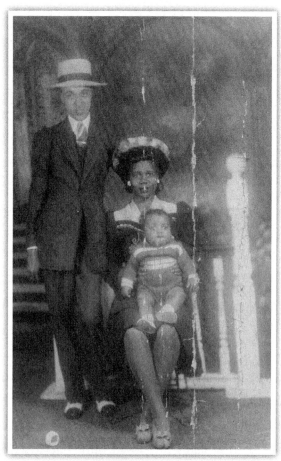

Milton Augustus Hawkins and Ernestine Blondine Hawkins (my mother and father) with my brother Bobby Hawkins when he was a baby.

I loved my mother very much and wanted to be just like her. I would mimic everything she did and to this day everyone says I am indeed my mother's child. She was nicknamed

"Babe" and you would not believe she had 6 children if you looked at her. My mother was beautiful and had a small waist, nice hips and legs and a beautiful smile. "Mum," as we called her, loved to dress and made certain that we were neat and clean at all times. I loved my mother very much, maybe too much, because I was jealous thinking she loved the others more than me. I especially thought she loved my oldest sister the best and as a result of that, I was always getting into trouble at home and I do mean ALWAYS getting in trouble, and constantly getting a spanking (in my time, we called it a beating). I was a needy child and just wanted my parents attention and affection. However, when you have six children and you are trying to make ends meet, it was hard to spread the love evenly.

We lived in a row home three stories high. Our family had the first two levels of the home and my grandmother had the third level. I was my grandmother's girl, but I really wanted the love from my mother. One day, I was being bad as usual, and I must have gone too far, because my grandmother told my mother, "Give her to me." I don't know what I did, but it must have been the last straw. On that day, I was sent upstairs to live with my grandmother. I called my grandmother "My Moo" and I actually loved being with her. My Moo taught me how to crochet and I would go out with her to sell the things she made. In addition, I spent a lot of time with her and she taught me good manners, how to act more respectful, and how to act like a lady. However, by being with my grandmother most of the time, I never really learned how to cook or scrub floors. Shep did a lot of the housework over the years but now I pay to have someone come clean my house for me. I guess I have My Moo to thank for that. ☺

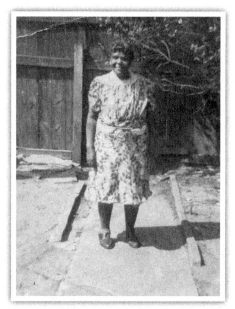

Henrietta Smith (My Grandmother/"My Moo")

During the day, I would come downstairs and play with Dim. Boy, she and I would have so much fun! Unfortunately, I never really played with Dee, who was three years older than me, because she was like a mother to all of us. During my time, parents had the oldest child take care of their brothers and sisters, and that was just the way it was. We never fought or argued with Dee, we just did what she told us to do. To this day, I still respect and listen to her advice.

When my sisters started school, I wanted to go with them, but unfortunately I was too young. I cried all day waiting for them to come home. When school was out, I would run to Dim and hug her and tell her how much I wanted to go to school with her. Dim and I really bonded together when she was 5 and I was 4. We were like two peas in a pod. One day, we were walking in a square where there was pretty green grass and flowers. I noticed a sign that said, "Seeded, keep off the grass." I looked at Dim and said, "I'm going to walk on this mother — grass." She looked at me in surprise and asked me where I had learned that word. I just laughed and told her that I didn't know. I must have heard it somewhere because I was only 4 years old, but I remember that time quite clearly. I must have also liked how I felt when I said that word because I kept wanting to say it over and over. Dim told me she was going to tell Mum on me, and I begged her not to. I knew what I was going to get if she told. I begged and begged and she finally agreed not to tell. I then asked her if we could seal it with our pinky fingers and we did. That was how we started sealing things, with our pinky fingers. True to her word, she never told on me. Unfortunately that day started my cussing career. When no one was around I said all kinds of bad words.

When I was finally old enough to go to school, I did not care too much about school work. The only class I did love was music class, and when I was six years old the teacher taught us this song which I still sing to all my little nieces:

"Shall we play we're lovely ladies all dressed up to go to parties

In our shining silver slippers and our crimps and feathered fans

There'll be candles, there'll be music, there'll be lots of cakes and candies

In and out we'll all go dancing just as lively as we can."

I would daydream about that song all the time because that was just what I wanted to do.

At age 11, my cousin Vernon gave me a boys 2-wheel bike and my father painted it for me so it looked pretty. How I enjoyed riding my bike, and would ride it only in the alley behind our house. While riding, I would call out to my mother each time I was on the bike and say, "Look Mum, no brakes!" My Mum would come to the window each time and tell me to stop it. I did this a lot of times and what I now realize is that I was crying "wolf" and didn't even know what I was doing. The story I am about to share has a couple of life lessons that I hope you are able to see. Unfortunately, I learned these lessons the hard way. It is my hope that each of you won't have to have a bad situation like mine happen before you learn the lesson God was trying to teach.

This one particular morning in May, I yelled it out again, "Look Mum, no brakes!" She was busy and didn't have any time for my antics so she said, "Stop worrying me!" However, when I went to apply the brakes this time, I REALLY didn't have any brakes. I screamed to my mother and she thought I was playing again so she didn't pay any attention to me. I went down that hill so fast and couldn't get off the bike in time. There was a car coming, and the next thing I knew, "WHAM!" A car hit me, and I was thrown up in the air and landed on the ground. I remember my mother running down the hill screaming. The driver of the car that hit me, picked me up and with him trying to put me in the car, my left ankle got shut up in the car door. I remember screaming in excruciating pain! (I was having a really bad day wasn't I?) I was rushed to John Hopkins Hospital and put in a cast all the way up to my thigh. Boy was I in pain! I can't describe how bad it was but take my word for it, it was really, really painful. After that incident I was told I would never be able to run, wear heels or do any kind of sports because of my injury. When my cast was taken off, I walked with a limp. It turns out that my injury healed incorrectly and my left leg became shorter than my right leg and that caused me to limp. My mother tried to help me get rid of that limp, so she would sit with me and make me walk around like a model so I could concentrate on trying not to limp. She also spoke words of encouragement and told me that I could overcome that limp. Her suggestion was for me to switch and move that leg slowly. From that day after the cast was removed I walked switching and I never stopped. This is why after that accident, I never exercised. As for the lessons, did you catch them? One lesson is that words have power. Be careful what you speak out of your mouth. I kept saying that I didn't have any brakes and guess what happened? I didn't have any. I kept crying wolf and then when I really needed help, no one believed me. I learned these two lessons quickly from this terrible accident and have tried to speak positive words of affirmation into the atmosphere as well as never cry wolf along my life journey. Those were two lessons well learned.

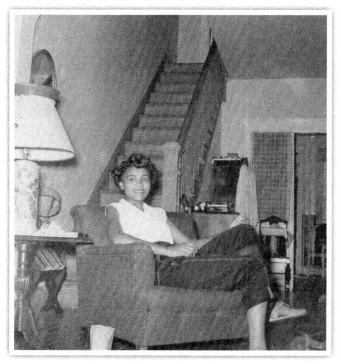

My younger years.

When I was around 12, I noticed my mother looking strange to me and I wasn't sure what was going on. I asked Dim what was wrong with her, and she told me that Mum was going to have another baby. I screamed, cussed and cried because then I knew I would never, ever get the love I wanted from my mother. I was so happy being called the "baby girl" and I didn't want that to change. I actually hated my mother and father for doing that to me, because having another baby meant I was no longer the one getting all the attention, and

I didn't like it one little bit. I got a beating every day for being bad. I really acted a fool, and instead of winning my mother's love and affection, I was actually pushing her away. Well, one day, along came the baby girl and I swore I would never look at her. Dim would hug me and tell me everything would be alright. How I wished I could be more like Dim, but I just couldn't be happy that this new baby was now in all of our lives. Time passed and still I was so angry about this new little person that had come and disrupted my life and knocked me out of my "baby girl" spot. More time passed, probably months, and I held fast to my resolve of not looking at that baby. Then one day, I felt a tugging at my heart and decided I would take a peek at my baby sister. The moment I saw her, I instantly fell in love with that little face. She was named Bernice but we all called her "Bunny". I loved her dearly from that day until this one.

I graduated from school in June, 1954 at the age of 17, and I decided I wanted to be a nurse because my cousin Ret was one. I also knew my family did not have money to send me to nursing school because my sister Dim was having a tough time with finances attending Coppin State, and this college was very inexpensive. Not only that, I knew I wasn't smart enough so I decided I wouldn't go to college. There's that low self-esteem rearing its ugly head again. Who told me I wasn't smart enough or good enough to go to college? No one ever said these things to me, this was the view that I had about myself and thus the reason I didn't go. If I had it to do all over again, I might have made a different choice. For everyone reading this book, I hope you are learning from some of my past mistakes. That negative self-talk will stop you in your tracks every time and you never want to miss out on opportunities that will help you go to another level in life because of fear, or those negative voices that swirl around in all of our heads.

Dim did struggle to make ends meet while she was in Coppin and since I had decided not to go to college, I made it my personal business to help her out financially in any way that I could. When she needed money for books, I told her to come with me and not say anything. There was a pool hall on Gay Street that we would pass from time to time. I told her that I was going in there and if I didn't come out in 15 minutes then she was to come in and get me. She didn't want me to go and tried to stop me. However, I reassured her that the men in the pool hall loved to hear me sing and do a little dance for them. Believe it or not, not one man put their hands on me. I would go in and do my song and dance, they would give me money and I turned around and gave it to my sister. Going in that pool hall again reminded me of a situation that happened when I was just a child that brought my life full circle.

You see, I was a pro at getting money from older men. At age six, I had an uncle who liked to drink and he never had any money, so he took me to a bar and would stand me on a table and have me sing. The song I sang was:

"Set them up Joe, we gotta make dough,

Make mine straight from the shoulder,

Let the cash box ring, ting-a-ling-a-ling,

With your hands in your pocket,

And your foot on the rail,

Set em up, fill em up… Joe!"

After I sang that song, the men would fall all over themselves to give me money. All the men thought I was cute doing my little song and dance and they just threw money my way. However, when I got the money, I would in turn just give it to my uncle. My sister told my Mum, I got a beating and could never see that uncle again. I did love my uncle and he never let anything happen to me. He said he loved me and that was all that mattered and all I wanted to hear.

Looking back on that situation, I know my mother was scared for her child. Anything could have happened to me in that pool hall. Thankfully nothing ever did. However, not only was my mother scared for me, but I also realized that my uncle was actually "pimping me out" to sing for the men, and then HE got all the money. No wonder my mother was so upset about that situation. In spite of our rocky relationship when I was growing up, she really did love me and cared about my well-being.

After graduating from high school in June, the summer went by fast and then September came. I saw all my friends going off to college and there I was still continuing working as a cashier at a Super Market. The realization of me not going to college had finally hit me, and I cried for about a week. Then one day I finally got myself together and just decided I had no choice and made the best of working there.

Even though I had made peace with the fact that I wasn't going to college, I was very, very sad for awhile because it appeared I had no real future. I mean, let's face it, I was a cashier, and that wasn't a career. I knew deep down that I couldn't stay in that job the rest of my life, and I had to figure out my next step and I had to figure it out soon. I am a firm believer that God always has a plan for his children, and whether I knew it or not, it was in his plan that I be right where I was in order for me to meet a special man.

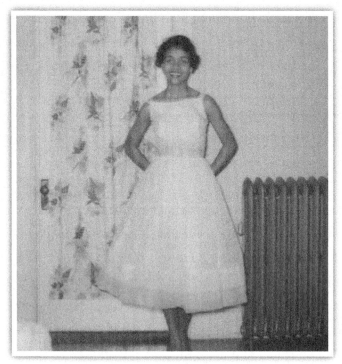

My days working as a cashier.

While working at the supermarket, a tall good-looking guy would come in to buy groceries. He would look at me and smile but he thought I was married because I wore a lot of rings. Dim had gotten married in 1955 and her husband owned a barber shop across from where I was working. Unbeknownst to me, this handsome man asked my brother-in-law if I were married and he told him that I wasn't married and that he should go after me. Well this guy had just bought a 1956 Plymouth and one day he came into the store, as we were closing, and asked me if he could take me home. Well as bad as I was, I would never have gotten into a strange man's car, so I quickly told him no thank you. This man wouldn't take no for an answer, so he drove slowly behind me and ended up following me home. I was a little concerned at first because I didn't know this guy and now he knew where I lived. My concerns faded away when I found out that my cousins knew him. Ever so slowly, I felt comfortable enough to start talking to this young man. He ended up meeting my parents, my sisters and my brothers too. Guess what? Everyone loved him.

After we had been talking and getting to know each other for awhile, he told me he worked at Western Electric and that he could put in a good word for me to get me hired there. True to his word, he pulled a few strings and I went to Western Electric to take a speed test to work in the factory. I wish I could tell you that everything went great but unfortunately it did not. I ended up failing the test because I was too slow. However, the people really liked me and told me to practice with match sticks and come back again to retake the test. Well I went home and practiced and practiced and when I felt like I had gotten a little faster, I went back and retook the test. This time I passed with flying colors! I was so happy because I was going to be making $1.26 per hour and I could finally help my parents financially. Don't laugh at my

$1.26 an hour salary because that was good money back in those days. I was just thankful that I was no longer working as a cashier and that I now had a job that I could grow and possibly make into a career.

While I worked at Western Electric, my best friends there were Edwina Weaver and Mildred Burroughs. I was such a shy, nervous and scared person when I first started working there, that it was almost comical. All I ever knew was being with my sister Dim, and I was also very sheltered. Because of this, I took that into my adulthood. People would say unkind things to me and I would cry. My friend Edwina told me that I needed to toughen up, but I didn't know how so I would just cry and cry. However, one day, a person said something mean to me and I was ready to cry and my friend Edwina, who called me "buddy" said, "Buddy, you had better NOT cry. Defend yourself!" I was scared but I jumped up and said, "Do you want to fight, because I do!" The person looked at me and backed down. She told me she didn't want to fight because it wasn't worth it. My friend Edwina was so proud of me for standing up for myself. She said, "See, people only sell wolf tickets. When you stand up for yourself, it takes away their power." From then on Edwina would call me "Rock," and when people saw I was no longer a cry baby, they left me alone. Then my friend Mildred helped me start dressing better and dressing more stylish. I was also finally starting to build up my self confidence. One thing most ladies will agree with is if you look good, you feel good. Can I get an Amen? If you wear clothes that look good on you, it can be a real self-esteem booster. I want to go on record to let you know that my confidence and self-esteem were at an all time high the more stylish I dressed. With Mildred's help, I was dressing better, looking better and feeling better. I credit both Edwina and Mildred for helping me develop, grow, change and learn how to be more comfortable around people as well as in my own skin. To this day, Edwina and I are still best friends. Unfortunately, Mildred died, but I will never forget all she taught me, and I thank God for her friendship.

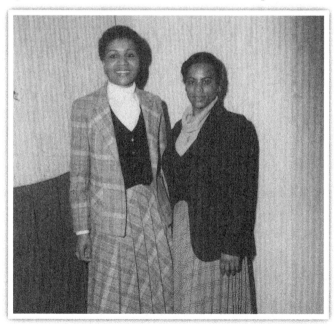

My friend Edwina Weaver and me during my days I worked at Western Electric.

There was another friend who also worked with us at Western Electric. His name was Mack Hardison, and he was always a good friend to me and my family and supported me in all my endeavors.

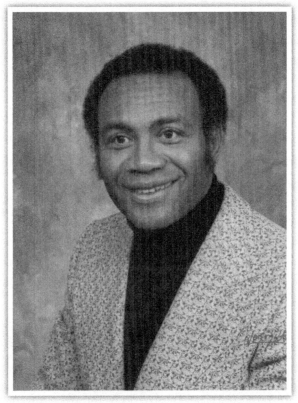

Collin J. Shepherd (The love of my life)

Now that I had more self-confidence I did get a little wild, but Dim told me I should settle down and get married. Remember the handsome friend that I started talking to and he ended up helping me get the job at Western Electric? Well my friend's name was Collin J. Shepherd. After my conversation with Dim, I decided it was indeed time for me to get married. So guess what I did? I went to Collin and asked HIM to marry ME. He smiled and said yes. I know most of you are in shock but yes it is true, I asked my husband to marry me, which was unheard of back in my day. I was ahead of my time. Somehow, that shy girl with the low self-esteem went away and a confident young woman emerged.

$\mathscr{C}$hapter 2
Shep and Michael –
The Two Loves Of My Life

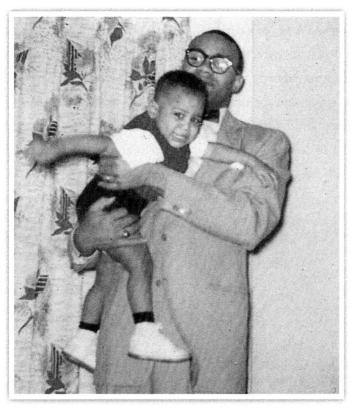

My husband and son in the early days.
Photo credit: Ernestine Shepherd

To be quite honest, my family was afraid for me to marry because I had gotten so wild, but we went ahead with our plans anyway. Collin started attending the same church with me and I sang in the choir. My parents went to the minister and asked him if we could be married in the church and he said that we could. We made sure we went to marital counseling classes and finally the big day arrived and we were married on November 25, 1956. Take a look at a few of our wedding pictures. It seems like yesterday when I walked down the aisle and said "I do", but I know it was a very long time ago. For those doing the math, you calculated correctly, we will be celebrating our 60th wedding anniversary this November! To God Be The Glory for keeping us together all these years! I called my husband Shep and he was and still is a good man. He also allowed me to help my parents with whatever they needed and I truly adore him for his kindness and quiet strength.

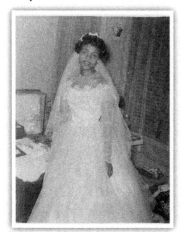

Here I am on my wedding day. What a beautiful day it was!

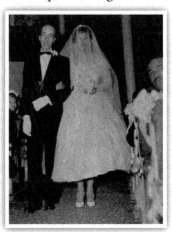

My father and me walking down the aisle.

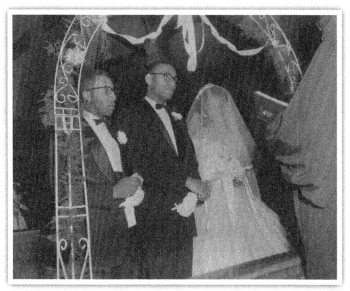

Collin and I reciting our wedding vows.

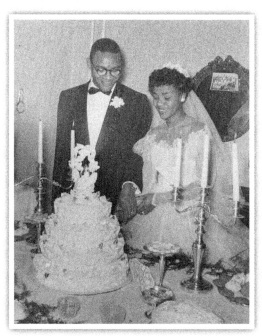

My husband and I cutting our wedding cake.
We were so happy!

After we were married, we found a small apartment inside a house. The people who owned the house lived on the first floor and we lived on the second floor. Somehow, someway, God has always been there for me even though I was not always the best person in the world. That is what you call favor.

We ended up moving into the home of a Methodist Minister, Rev. S.W. Fields and his lovely wife Dolly Fields. They took us in as their children and treated us well. Mrs. Dolly found out that I could not cook, and every day we came home from work, dinner was on the table for us. In addition, they kept us grounded and we had prayer all the time.

I had only been married 3 months before I became pregnant. Boy we didn't wait long did we? ☺ When I found out I was pregnant, I was still working at Western Electric and making good money. I was very upset and frightened when I found out I was going to have a child. During those first few months I was so sick that I had to take medication. I never gained any more than 14 lbs during the entire 9 months I was pregnant! Yikes! Now that I put this on paper, that was pretty bad right? The little bit of food I did keep down was going to nourish the baby, but not me. In addition, I was really sick the entire time I was pregnant.

People on my job didn't help either. They frightened me by saying I might be pregnant in my tubes since I wasn't gaining any weight. I had never heard of that before and I got so scared. I told my husband that I never wanted to get pregnant again. The constant stress, strain and worry for my baby's health was just a little bit too much for me, and I really meant what I said about not getting pregnant again. I just couldn't go through it again. For those who were wondering why I only got pregnant that one time and that one time only, that was the reason why.

Towards the end of my pregnancy I was feeling better, and felt like my old self. I was out and about as normal and almost forgot I was pregnant. ☺ Every Halloween, my oldest sister Dee would have a party at her house for just the family. My parents, my sister Velvet, her husband and daughter Dietra were there. Dee, at that time, had only one child, Teresa, and they were there. In addition my baby sister Bern was just ten years old and she was there too. On October 31, 1957, we were there for our annual party. Boy we were having a good time dancing and jumping around. My mother kept telling me not to jump around so much or I may have my baby there. I was feeling so good and I didn't listen. I just kept on jumping and dancing. When the party was over I felt very strange. I can't describe it, I just felt weird. My family all laughed and told Shep I would be in the delivery room that night. Well I didn't go that night but I sure was there that next morning. My mother was right, all that jumping actually put me into labor and Michael was born November 1, 1957, on a Friday morning at 7:30 am. I was happy that I had a boy because I really had made up my mind that I did not want to go through that ever again. I was firm on that decision and Shep respected my feelings on that issue.

My husband called Michael his prize package and his pride and joy. I vowed that I would always show him I loved him and tried all I could to make him happy. He had two of everything, but we made sure he was not spoiled. My son was always being prayed over. Rev. Fields and Dolly Fields prayed for him every day. When we would leave for work they prayed over him, when we came home they prayed for him. I truly believe prayer changes things and that is why God has always been there for Michael through his life because of the constant prayer we bathed him in since he was a baby. When Michael was young I called him Beau, Beau. Then later Beau and now finally Mike.

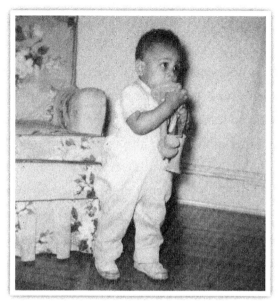

Michael at one years old.

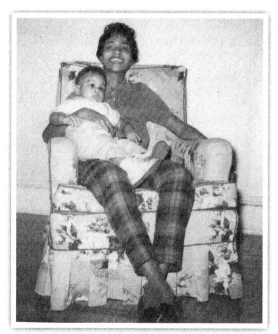

Michael and me just relaxing.

I always kept Michael in matching yellow sleepers, booties, blankets and sheets. He had a yellow bassonet as well. I also would hold and kiss him all the time and I cried and cried when it was time for me to return to work because I didn't want to leave him. I know some of you are thinking I was smothering him with affection, and I probably was, but I couldn't help it. I was determined to show my son love, and I did. It is so interesting how the things we didn't feel we got as children or things we didn't get enough of growing up, we try to make up for in our children and that is exactly what I did with Michael. I hope he understands that everything I did was out of my love and concern for him and even if he didn't quite understand why his mother was so affectionate and loving, there was an underlying reason why I was and still am.

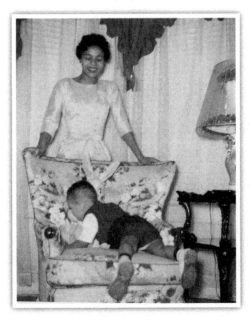

Michael and me.

Rev. Fields christened Michael at his church and we were there every Sunday. I could not ask for anything more, a good husband and a wonderful son. I do realize now that sometimes I went overboard with my love and affection, but Michael grew up to be a fine young man. No one could believe I had changed so much. I was a good wife and a good mother. I loved and still love my son and husband very much.

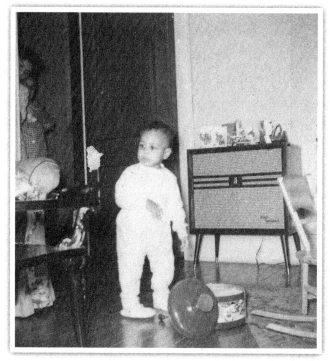

Michael in the early years.

Being a new mother wasn't easy at first, but I was so glad that my sister Dim was nearby. She and I called each other daily because we lived a couple blocks from each other. However, the thing I was most pleased about during the days of my early motherhood was when the unthinkable happened! My mother and I actually bonded! Can you believe it? Finally, the thing I had longed for and prayed for had finally happened and it was like heaven! My mother and I would go to church together and Dim would come along with us. I was also able to have beautiful clothes made for my mother and was also able to spend a lot of quality time with her. My husband was so happy to see that I finally had the love of my mother. When Dim and I started our exercise program, my mother came along for awhile. I am convinced that the birth of my son brought my mother and me closer together and I loved him all the more for that.

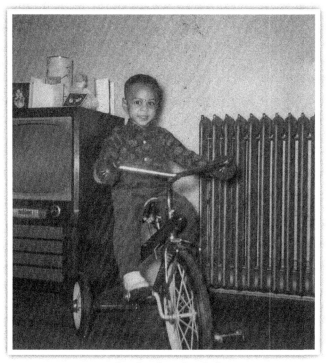

Michael riding his bike.

I remember when Michael was little, he loved to ride his bike. He would ride it up and down the street all the time and he could do all kinds of tricks on it as well. Later on he wanted a mini bike and we bought it for him. However, one day, the unimaginable happened. He got hurt really bad on his bike and ruptured his spleen. He fell off his bike really hard, and although I knew he scraped himself pretty bad, I didn't realize how bad it was. I probably didn't think anything was wrong because he came inside as he normally did and went to bed. In the middle of the night he got up to go to the bathroom, but when he went to the bathroom he saw a lot of blood in the toilet. Luckily he got me up, I saw the blood and immediately rushed him to the hospital. It turned out he had to have emergency surgery. Oh my goodness! I shudder to think what would have happened had Michael just gone and laid back down after he saw that blood. I thank God every day that he had the presence of mind to immediately come get me when he saw the blood. He ended up being in the hospital for months and after he was released, it took several more months for him to get completely back on track. God is good and I truly thank Him for being there for my son when he needed him the most. I am a witness that God is truly a healer!

After Michael graduated from high school and entered into college, we knew it would be a new experience for him. We prayed that all the values and guidance we had taught him would stay with him and he would remember them when times got tough. We taught him to be kind and gentle with people, treat others like you wanted to be treated and forgive others.

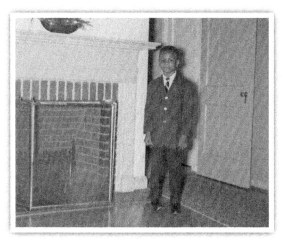

Michael at age 8.

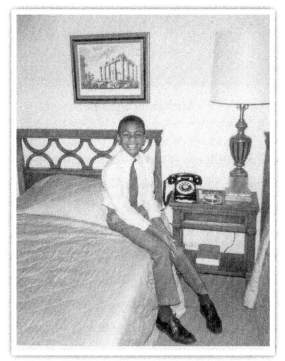

Michael on his way to church.

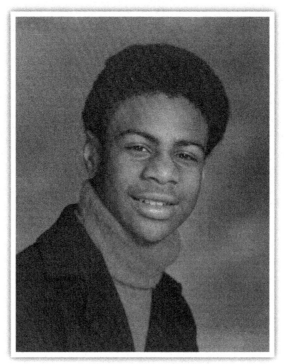

Michael at age 14.

Michael loved to play sports. You name the sport and he loved to play it. However, baseball and basketball were his favorites, and Shep and I believe sports helped develop his leadership skills. When I look back over Michael's life, I see a quiet, reserved and kind young man. He made some mistakes, and had his share of setbacks, but he also had many bright spots and achievements along the way. One of his biggest obstacles to overcome was his addiction to alcohol, which was very detrimental to him. He had some dark days, and it wasn't easy, but by the grace of God and support from Shep and me, his sponsor and AA support groups, he was able to overcome this addiction. To God be the glory!

The Ageless Journey of Ernestine Shepherd Continues...

Chapter 3

The Journey Into Fitness

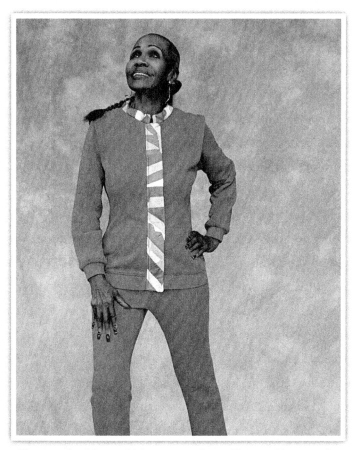

Photo credit: Maynard Manzano – Magic Glamour Photography

As I mentioned before, my husband Shep is the Chairman of the Trustee Board at Union Memorial United Methodist Church. I am proud to say that Shep, Michael and I have been members for over 50 years. Each summer some organizations would have cook outs in conjunction with our church. This particular summer, my husband told us about a cook out with some of the members. We were going to Carolyn and Joseph Boston's summer home, and what a lovely home they had. Shep said we should bring our bathing suits because they had a large swimming pool. We had not worn bathing suits in years so we had to go buy them. We were so excited to buy the suits and we went to Owings Mills to a store called Gantos. There were so many beautiful bathing suits there and I was ready to try them on. I grabbed 3 suits, a 1-piece and two 2-piece suits. I really didn't know what size so each one was a different size. My sister did the same thing. She and I got the same style but in different colors. We were both happy and I was talking loud and saying I could hardly wait to go to the cookout to show off my bathing suit. However my sister, who was very quiet, just looked at me and laughed. I started softly singing because I was excited and happy, but my sister never said a word. We started with the 2-piece suit. Mine was a hot red and hers was black. We put them on and I looked in the mirror and stopped singing. My sister looked at me and started laughing. I got angry and said, "What is so funny?" She said, "Teeny, when in the world did your thighs and hips get THAT big?" I told her that they must have come from me wearing a girdle that stopped on my thighs and that is why I had dents in them. That is really what I thought when I saw all those dents on my thighs. In addition, wearing clothes and not really looking at my thighs, I never thought about those thighs anymore.

No one saw my thighs except for Shep, and he thought that was the way thighs looked at age 56. ☺ Even though I had big thighs, I was still small waist up. After my sister examined me, I looked at her and said, "Wait a minute, what in the world happened to you?" She had always been larger than me but not anymore. I was really surprised by her legs because they were so small. I just could not believe what I saw. I thought to myself that clothes really can hide a multitude of things. I actually cried a little looking at her because I thought she was sick being so small, and I didn't know what to think about myself with my thighs looking so big.

My sister told me not to try on anymore suits and just to put them back on the rack. She then informed me that we needed to get our bodies back in shape by exercising. We didn't buy any suits that day. Instead, we purchased long pants and tops and left the store.

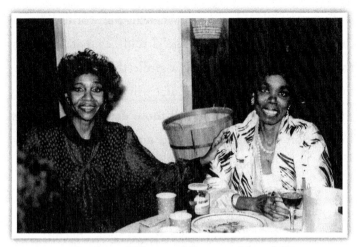

**Check out Velvet and I at age 56 and 57
before we started on our fitness journey.**

After leaving the store we sat in the car in disbelief. We didn't realize the change in our bodies. Mine, I needed to tone and get that mess out of my thighs. Hers, she needed to build up because she was too small. I did ask her how she lost all that weight in her lower body and I hadn't even noticed. I also wondered how I really thought all the dimples and junk on my legs were due to wearing a girdle. My sister said it again that we needed to find some place to go to tone up our bodies. I told her that she was 57 and I was 56, did she really think exercise would make a change? She told me that we should at least give it a shot. I wanted to know where and when we would begin and she told me that we would find a place and begin soon. We hugged and put our pinky fingers together and she said, "Is it a deal?" I said yes and our journey into fitness actually started there because we spoke out what we were going to do and did so with intention.

When we arrived back home, Shep said, "So girls, let me see the bathing suits you bought." We laughed and told him the story, and then showed him the outfits we bought. He told us that if we were happy and were still going to the cookout, then he was happy too.

We did indeed go to the cookout and I wore navy blue pants and a white top and my sister wore black pants and a blue top. We weren't dressed to get in the pool but we at least looked good nonetheless. The cookout, as I mentioned, was held at Carolyn and Joe Boston's summer home and boy was it a breathtakingly, beautiful place! A few names of people there I remember were Glyndi Johns and his wife, Ellen C. Johns, as well as Donald Atkinson and his wife Rosemary Atkinson. Glyndi and Donald were swimming in the pool with the others and everyone looked as though they were having so much fun splashing around in the water. How I wished we were in there with them. As we sat by the pool with other people and just talked, Rosemary mentioned she was exercising at a college. My sister immediately perked up and wanted to know what college and what the cost was for the class. She told us that she was exercising at Coppin College (the name has changed now) and said there was a good instructor there. That very next week, we went to sign up for the exercise class. Just like that, with one quick decision, the journey had officially begun... the journey that I have been on for years and am still on as of this writing. That journey is the journey into fitness.

Chapter 4
My Sister Dim –
Her Life and Her Vision

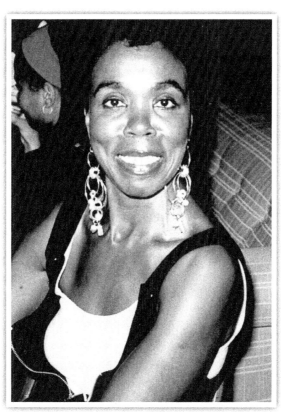

My sister Mildred (Dim/Velvet) Hawkins.
Photo credit: Ernestine Shepherd

THE LOCATION OF THE GYM WAS CLOSE to our home and we could walk there if we wanted to. We immediately signed up to start this fitness journey. We signed up not knowing what to expect and had no idea what we were doing, but we knew we had to get fit. We made a decision and then took action. That is the only way you are going to start on your own journey. You have to make a decision to start, just as we did.

The instructor was Jay Bennett and we went up to introduce ourselves. He asked us what we were expecting to get out of the class. My sister said she wanted to tone and build up her body because she had gotten so small and wanted to know if he could help her. He smiled and told her that he could. He then asked me the same question. I told him I wanted to tone my upper body and get the mess out of my thighs, but wanted my hips to stay the same size because I loved my hips. He told me it didn't work that way. No spot retouching around here. My sister told me to just keep quiet and take the class. She reminded me of the promise we made in the car and I told her I hadn't forgotten.

Jay told us to wear something comfortable that we can move around in and some tennis shoes. He also told us to stay and watch him teach his class. He taught aerobics and weight training classes and we ended up staying and watching aerobics class for the entire hour. After we left, I told my sister that

I didn't believe I would be able to hang because I never did any exercising because of my broken ankle that I had at age 12.

She told me that now that I was 56 my ankle should be healed. I said the doctor told me I would never be able to do any jumping around again. She then said these words: "You also told me that the doctor said you would never be able to wear heels again either and you do. So keep quiet, you ARE going to do it." Guess what I did? I got myself geared up and ready to take the journey with her into fitness. Did you notice all the excuses I was making? Have any of you made excuses like that and can't seem to get started? Thank God that Dim was my accountability partner and she didn't pay any mind to any of my excuses. She kept me on task and sometimes that is what you need to stay the course. Take my advice and make a decision to just do it and then take action and begin. If you can, get an accountability partner that can push you and keep you on track with your goals.

We ended up buying 3 new exercise outfits each, which were one piece suits that were identical, only in different colors. We both also wore white tennis shoes and we just knew we looked good. ☺ When we went to our first class Jay called my sister Blackwell and me Shepherd. The class was full of men and women and after the warm up, he played a song called, "I got the power". They all started jumping around doing aerobics and my sister jumped right in with them. I tried but quickly got tired. I was out of shape! However, I did what I could the first day. That is key, even though I couldn't do everything, I at least did something. We both did a lot of sweating, but it really was fun. What I noticed was each time we went it got better and better, and much easier, but I wasn't completely putting my all into it like my sister was. She was focused and practiced being determined, dedicated and disciplined to be fit right away. I was just there because I promised her I would be.

When Jay Bennett didn't teach class, Edna Simmons taught. That lady could really go! She also did a lot of things to help each person. I really loved working out with both of them. My sister was doing great because she did not have to lose weight like I did so it did not take long to see a change in her. But trying to get my legs toned was tough and I complained all the time. When you got good in the class you could go on the front line and work out. Well, guess who was on the front line and who wasn't? LOL One thing I did love to do was dress up. My sister and I would both wear some beautiful clothes to exercise in. Everyone would wait to see what we would wear next. I was such a show off. LOL The dressing up was fun for me.

One day, Jay told us that we needed to start lifting weights. My sister was happy, but I told him that I wasn't going to do it because I did not want to look like a man. Jay assured us we wouldn't look like a man and we would only be toning up. I followed Dim's lead and started lifting weights. At first I could not lift a 2 lb weight, but she could. Even though I wanted to give up, I stayed. Again, I saw an immediate change in her after she started lifting consistently, but of course…not me. Everyone started making comments about how good my sister was starting to look because of her consistent weight lifting but I didn't compliment her. One night at the gym I got so angry that I ended up walking out and walked home. I told myself that I would never return.

Later, my sister came to my house after she noticed I was no longer at the class. She asked why I left and I told her I was a little jealous of all the attention she was getting and my body wasn't changing. She hugged me and told me how much she loved me and asked me to come back, work hard and I too would look the same. She said, "promise?" and I told her yes. Then we sealed the deal like we always did with our pinky fingers. She told me that we were in this together and I couldn't give up. I went back to the gym as I promised her and worked hard and actually began to really enjoy it.

One day my sister told me that we should try to inspire and motivate others to live a healthy, positive and confident life by eating correctly, drinking plenty of water, doing strength training, some type of cardio, but most of all through prayer because you cannot do anything without prayer. She said we would then call it our ministry. I hollered out, "Mission." She replied, "No, this is our MINISTRY." So I agreed. She told me the plan and below is what she laid out:

1. Change our names
2. Change our hair style
3. Dress alike only in different colors
4. Develop a mantra
5. Find a creed
6. Always have a smile on our faces and mean it
7. Give everyone a hug and mean it
8. Don't talk bad about anyone
9. Practice what we preach about healthy eating
10. Be strong and don't get upset if someone doesn't like what we say or how we look

She named a few more things and I agreed. We sealed it again with our pinky fingers and we were on our way to implementing the plan. She came up with our mantra which is: "Determined, Dedicated and Disciplined to Be Fit."

I thought the plan was great but I asked her to please not tell me I couldn't wear my long nails or that I couldn't wear all my make up because I liked doing that. She didn't have a problem with that. I did agree to change my hair color from blond to black so we could both match. Speaking of hair color, we used a black rinse in our hair and we were exercising one day and started sweating. I looked at her and noticed the sweat that was running down was black! I fell out laughing and she asked what I was laughing about and I told her that her black rinse was running. Little did I know that mine was running too. That was the day we decided to stop using the black rinse in our hair. We just let the color wear out.

My sister also found the right creed that said the things that matched what we were trying to aspire to be and do. It was and still is a beautiful and powerful creed, but I told her I didn't know if I could do it for the following reasons:

1. I am not strong
2. I like to talk about people
3. I am not hugging everyone

I kept naming all the things I could NOT do and that's when she told me that this is where prayer comes in. I just said, "Oh really?" She then told me to read the creed once each day because the more I read it, the more I would follow it. I told her I would indeed read it. On the next page is the creed she chose and it is one I read every single day:

I Promise Myself...

To be so strong that nothing can disturb my peace of mind.

To talk health, happiness, and prosperity to every person I meet.

To make all my friends feel that there is something worthwhile in them.

To look at the sunny side of everything and make my optimism come true.

To think only the best, to work only for the best, and to expect only the best.

To be just as enthusiastic about the success of others as I am about my own.

To forget the mistakes of the past and press on to the greater achievements of the future.

To wear a cheerful expression at all times and give a smile to every living creature I meet.

To give so much time to improving myself that I have no time to criticize others.

To be too large for worry, too noble for anger, too strong for fear, and too happy to permit the presence of trouble.

To think well of myself and to proclaim this fact to the world, not in loud words, but in great deeds.

To live in the faith that the whole world is on my side, so long as I am true to the best that is in me.

(Christian D. Larson - 1912)

Being optimistic isn't always easy. Most of us tend to focus on the negatives associated with our lives and our bodies and we need to just STOP IT! Have you considered that everything you do today, think about or even say is related to your future? I encourage you to read our mantra every day and focus on the positive and dump the negative thinking.

My sister and I were having so much fun exercising, dressing alike and just living a productive, healthy and peaceful life. People would stop us and ask us questions about exercising. Also at the gym, Jay Bennett would always have a Halloween party and we would wear costumes. We always won first place because we came up with such cute costumes. At one of the parties, we met a guy named Raymond Day (who we call Ray). Ray came dressed as a pirate and boy did he look good! We asked where he exercised and he said Capitol Fitness. We decided to start going to Capitol Fitness with our new names, she – Velvet and me – Magenta and that is how we signed up.

Here is a picture of Ray. See why we wanted to work out with him?

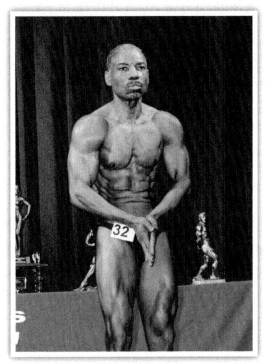

Raymond Day Body Building Picture

My sister told me to change Magenta to Ernie. At first Ray called me Magenta. We worked out with him 3 days a week and he taught us so much. He had done many body building shows and took us to many as well. That is when my sister said we would become body builders and try for the Guinness Book of World Records as 2 of the oldest sisters to be body builders. I just laughed. She told me not to laugh because anything was possible and we could even be in Ripley's Believe It Or Not. Ray told us to follow our dreams and never give up.

Ray had my sister doing heavy squats and lifting heavy weights, but I could not do as much as her. However, this time, I did not get angry. I just did what I could and was happy with that. We became three peas in a pod. I took Ray home to meet my husband and he became friends with my family. If anyone was determined, dedicated and disciplined to be fit, it was Ray and my sister, but I was doing my best to hang in there with them. We all ate healthy and overall took care of our health and well-being. We also would go out of town to Mr. Olympia and Arnold Classics and many other body building shows. I whispered to my sister when we saw Carla Dunlap compete and I asked her if she liked how she looked. She said that she did and that she wanted to look like her. Velvet started buying magazines or anything with Carla Dunlap on them. She especially liked her wearing shorts and sitting at the pull down machine and working her back. She had Ray give us a lot of exercises working our back muscles. We never looked like Carla, but we had a nice back. Everything was going just great and I was really enjoying working out now. But of course all good things sometimes must come to an end.

One day we were at the gym and Velvet said, "Teeny" (that is what she called me). She said, "You know I love you so much and we really make a great team. I am so proud of us. If anything would happen to me, could you still go on and fulfil our dream?" I quickly looked up and said, "What did you say?" She repeated it and I told her to stop being silly that we will be working together until the end. I reminded her about what we said as kids, that when we got really old, we were going to sit on her front porch and just rock. We said we were going to talk about how our children never gave us any trouble (that was a private joke ☺). I told her that we had to do that. She just grabbed my hand and looked in my face and repeated what she had said. I then asked her if something happened to me, could she keep going. She said, "Teeny, stop it and listen to me. Something is going to take me away very quickly." She had a grandson that she called "Lovie" and she loved him dearly. She would always say she was living for him. I reminded her about Lovie and told her that I didn't want to hear any more of that talk. Period, end of discussion.

She didn't mention it again for a while about something happening to her. I was overjoyed that she did not. At that time I worked as a manager at a Beauty mart store, and whenever I was on break I would call her. This one particular day when I called, she told me that her head had been hurting her every day for a while, and on that day it was hurting worse than ever. We wore our hair the same way and I told her that sometimes I would get a headache because my braid was pulled back too tight. I told her to open it and let it just hang loose. The next time she said she could not see out of one eye, but as the day went on, it had gotten a little better. Next, it felt like it was water running in her ears, and she got up and didn't know what was going on. My sister Bern called and asked what was going on because she noticed Dim (Velvet) was acting strange. I told her nothing was wrong, because I really thought she was going to be ok. Then Velvet told me she couldn't use her hands and that is when I got really nervous and told her I was going to call my parents and Bern. I found out that she had already contacted them and they were on their way to her house. I called back and she seemed ok. I told her the family was on the way and that I was happy because I didn't want her dying on me and leaving me lonely. She laughed and said she wasn't dying. However in a split second, she was talking strange again. I was not there when my parents and Bern arrived at her house, but apparently she couldn't open the door. They told her to throw the keys through the mail slot so they could get in. She finally was able to get the keys out to them so they could get in, and when they saw her, they knew she needed to get to the hospital immediately.

They took her to the hospital, but the wait was too long, so they were about to leave when I finally arrived. They decided to go to another hospital. I sat in the back seat of the car with her head in my lap and I was rubbing her head. I told her that when she got well I would tell her how she worried me. The only thing she said was, "Remember what we agreed." She then held out her pinky finger. I knew what she wanted me to do so we sealed it with our pinky fingers. I was nervous and wanted to cry but I held back my tears. When we arrived at the hospital she surprisingly was able to walk in. When they asked her what was wrong she said it was her head and she didn't know why it had to hurt so bad. They took her immediately, examined her and they found that she had a brain aneurysm. Unfortunately, it had already burst and that was the water she felt running in her ears. It was blood that she felt running, not water. They tried to save her, but to no avail. My beloved sister, who had always been there for me, died. Yes as kids we fussed but never fought. I could tell her anything, and she understood me better than I understood myself. I was devastated! I was deeply, totally and completely devastated that she was gone. I got up from my seat in the hospital and ran around saying, "I don't have anyone, I just don't have anyone!" My baby sister came to me and said, "You have me." I loved my baby sister very much but at that time, that was not what I wanted. I just cried and cried. On that Sunday morning I went down to

Mt. Zion United Methodist Church and sat on the back pew listening to the minister preach. I sat there and just cried and cried. I thought to myself, "How could God let this happen? She was a good person, never did any harm to anyone and always studied her bible with my mother. Here I sit not doing good things and God took her. I don't understand. Why? Why? Why?" These thoughts swirled around in my head for a long time. I finally left the church and went home still not hearing an answer to my questions.

My sister's service was held at Mt. Zion United Methodist Church and I managed to sing the Lord's Prayer and was able to listen to Reverend Brown give her eulogy. However, I was a total and complete mess and hurt all through that service. I don't know how I managed to make it through that day, but somehow I did. There was no burial or going to a cemetery, because Velvet was cremated.

I went home after her funeral and I hated everything, everyone, myself and especially God. Why did He allow this to happen. Remember all the bad words that I used to say? Well they were revived when this happened. I let them rip because I was so angry. Fortunately, Keith, Velvet's grandson she loved so dearly, ended up coming to stay with me for a short time.

Keith's mother's name was Dietra, and I made certain that her son got to school. I loved him so much because I knew just how much Velvet loved him. My husband would drive Keith to school each day and then go pick him up.

My way of trying to heal after Velvet's death was for me to write to her each day and tell her just what was going on. Some days I missed her so much that I could barely breathe. She was truly my best friend. Another way I tried to heal myself was being with her grandson. Even though Shep took Keith to school most of the time, I also took him sometimes as well. On days that I took Keith to school, however, I wanted to stay all day and the teacher permitted me to do so. I wanted to be close to him and make sure that he was safe. Once again, I was going overboard with my love and affection, but during that time I needed to do that to get through that very difficult time in my life. One day his teacher, Mrs. Perry, told me that I had to let him go. She told me I had to let him stand on his own two feet and be in class by himself. It hurt and I cried, but I did as she asked. The first day he cried because I wasn't going to be with him, but after that, he was a big boy and didn't cy any more.

I finally went back to work at my job managing the Beauty mart. I didn't want to go, but my husband thought it best for me to be around other people rather than being in the house acting mean and saying bad words. I hated going back to work, but I knew I had to try to heal my grieving heart, and get my life back on track.

My nerves were shot, I was depressed, had panic attacks and acid reflux. You name it, and I had it. I was known in the ER because when we would arrive at night, the nurses that were on duty would say, "Here comes Ernestine again, what brings you in this time?" My chest would be on fire and the room always felt like it was closing in on me. I hated the way I was living, but I didn't care because I knew living this way wouldn't be long and I could be with Velvet. I know I was being selfish, but my mind was not right. When I think back, I ask myself, "How could I have done that?" I loved my husband and son very much, but during that time, I was just out of it. My husband and son were good to me, but I was not good to them.

One night after tossing and turning, I finally drifted off to sleep. I can remember tossing and turning a little more and my eyes opened. Who did I see but Velvet standing there looking at me. I could not believe what I was seeing. I just stared at her in shock and disbelief. After looking at me for a moment, she began to speak very quietly and quickly to me. She said the following: "You are not doing what I asked you to do. You made a promise and you are not keeping it. Get up, stop feeling sorry for yourself and do what I asked you to do." I was ready to talk with her but as quickly as she appeared, that is how quickly she disappeared. I got up and looked around the room, but no one was there. Then I just sat there stunned for a few minutes. Was I dreaming or what? The next day I thought about what happened and I cried all day. By now you all can tell that I am a big crybaby right? Or rather I used to be. I'm a lot better now. ☺

That night I told my husband what happened. He said, "Now what do you plan to do? Are you going to stay in this funk and waste your life away or are you going to get up and try to keep the promise you made to your sister?" I got angry and didn't answer him. I just left the room and started crying again. I think a week went by and then one day, on a Friday morning, I got up, got dressed, left the house and went to a church I had never been to before. I sat in the back and listened to the choir singing. I listened to the scripture being read and I thought to myself that I wanted to get out of there. All of a sudden, the organist started playing a hymn that my sister and I liked and it was one I sang at my church. The words of the song are:

Here I am, Lord. Is it I Lord?
I have heard you calling in the night.

I will go, Lord, if you lead me.
I will hold your people in my heart.

Suddenly, the tears came to my eyes, and I heard this voice yell out very loud. Imagine my surprise when I realized it was my voice. I could not believe it as me, because nothing at church ever used to touch me that way. I could not stop. I stood up and said, "Restore to me the joy of my salvation! Restore to me the joy of each new day! Give me back the love I once had for you and never ever let me slip away!" How could I have done that? I don't know, but I did it. I used to see people at church doing what I did, but I thought they just wanted to be seen. Here I was in my fifties really getting the Holy Spirit. Me, who had made fun of everyone making all that noise. I was asked if I wanted to become a member of that church, but I said no.

You can't imagine how different I felt after that. I came home and I felt like a new person. I told my husband what happened and he hugged me and asked me what I planned to do next. He was worried that I would continue in my depressed state. However, I told him that I was going to fulfill my sisters dream and become a better person. Both he and my son told me that whatever I decided to do that they would be in my corner.

When I decided I was going to follow my sisters dream, my son gave me 4 DVD's of Sylvester Stallone in Rocky. I wondered why he gave them to me, but I watched all 4 DVD's anyway and ended up falling in love with Sylvester Stallone. I noticed all the problems he had in the Rocky movies, but he remained strong enough to overcome them.

After my son gave me those DVD's about the Rocky Balboa character, I was extremely inspired . Even though I know it was a movie, Sylvester Stallone really brought the Rocky character to life, and so many things in his films reminded me of my own struggles after my sister died. I liked what Stallone said, "It's not about how hard you get hit, but how you keep moving forward." That is how winning is done. The Rocky movies invoked a positive emotional state in me, and the dynamic music transforms me and makes me ready to take on the world. I pictured Rocky as a strong, well-developed person and I decided that I would try in some way to be like him. I saw how he would drink egg whites, so I started drinking them, and I still drink them to this day. I also saw how hard he would train for a fight, and I started working out hard.

Whenever I was down, I would play those DVD's, and anyone who has my cell number knows that the Rocky theme song plays as my ringtone. Sylvester Stallone has no idea the role he played in Rocky also played a big role in my life, and I appreciate him and hope one day to meet him.

Watching those DVD's that day is when I made a decision to go back to being determined, dedicated and disciplined to be fit for life. I had gotten off track, but was determined to come out of my depression and honor my promise to my sister, but most of all to myself.

$\mathcal{C}$hapter 5
Honoring My Promise To Carry On My Sisters Vision

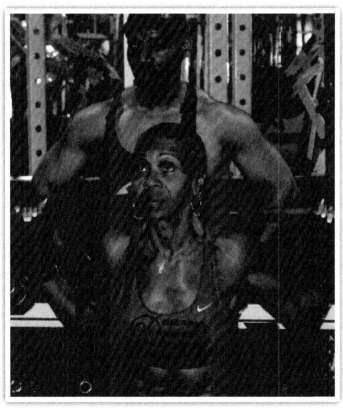

My second trainer, Raymond Day and me.
Photo credit: Ernestine Shepherd

I CALLED MY OLD FRIEND, RAYMOND DAY, who worked out with my sister and me, and told him I wanted to start working out again. I would get off work at 7 PM so I asked him if I took my work out clothes to work and changed there, would he take me to the gym? He said that he would and we began a routine. Every Monday, Wednesday and Friday I started going to the gym and working out with Ray. I never saw anyone so dedicated to working out! On days when I said I didn't want to go, he told me that we were going. He would always say to me, "Don't quit on being fit."

We trained hard. Ray then told me that I needed to get my diet right. It isn't just enough to exercise, you do indeed have to eat right as well. He knew a man by the name of Todd Swinney that was big in nutrition. In 1998, he took me to Todd who was and still is into sports nutrition. I told Todd I needed his help because even with all my working out, my thighs still weren't right. I told him that I didn't want to take supplements and he was able to design an eating program for me which I still follow to this day. I would go to him each month and as always, my upper body was fine; however, I was still fighting with my thighs. Eventually, with Todd's help, I was able to get my thighs under control.

One day Ray told me he was going to take a picture of me and send it to Essence Magazine. He said if they liked it then I would appear in their publication. I laughed and said, "Now Ray, you know they won't like my pictures." He didn't listen to me, thank God, and sent the picture anyway. Well guess what happened? They did indeed like my picture and asked me to come to New York for a photo shoot. In honor of my sister, I wore a black dress with T-straps that was her daughter Dietra's dress. I met Mikki Taylor, who worked for Essence Magazine, and I was so honored to have done my first real photo shoot at 62 years old. Check out my picture and what I wore.

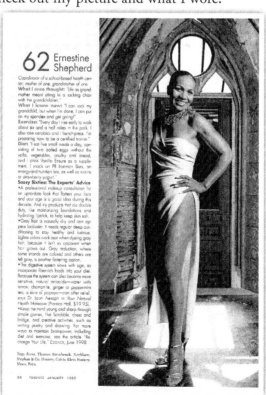

Ernestine Shepherd Essence Picture

To my surprise, everyone loved the photo shoot. I was talked about on many radio shows, TV and magazines. I was surprised, but humbled, and loved that the vision was starting to take off.

Mikki Taylor reached out to me again and asked me to come to New York because she was writing a book called "Self-Seduction" and she wanted me to be part of it. I went to New York again and the response was just as awesome, and many more TV and radio stations asked me to come for interviews. Ray then started taking me to local body building shows. This is when I discovered that I liked wearing really nice work-out clothes. I started purchasing clothes from different websites and people would just marvel at the different outfits that I came up with. We also traveled out of state to many professional body building shows and I met many body builders all over the world.

During this time, the Beauty mart was closing, and it was now time to get another job. Luckily, my sister Bern, hired me at her school. Unfortunately, because of my job change, my schedule changed as well. My schedule changed to the point I could no longer work out with Ray. To keep me on track, he introduced me to a man named Ernest Jones. Ray told me I would be in good hands with Ernest and I was.

Each day I would take my work-out clothes with me to the school and would change there and go to the gym that was close by. Ray kept in contact daily to keep up with my progress.

Ray and I would still go to body building shows. At one show I met a judge by the name of Sheritha Mckenzie. She was really fit and had won many body building trophies. She also had her own studio and looked great. I was impressed with her body definition and knew she worked really hard. One day she invited me to visit her studio called Bodies on Line. I liked how she trained people and I asked if I could become a trainer there. She told me I could and that was my first job as a trainer. Sheritha was very kind to me and taught me everything I needed to know about becoming a trainer. At the shows where she was a judge, she made certain I presented the trophies to the winners. I could never ever forget all she has done for me and I appreciate her very much.

One day out the blue Ray said, " When are you going to really do what your sister asked you to do?" I didn't say anything. He told me that it was time for me to go to a body building show in Washington, DC and that he wanted to introduce me to a man by the name of Yohnnie Shambourger who put on the show.

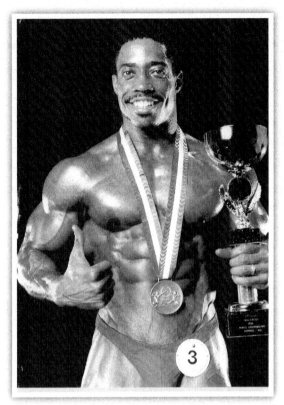

Yohnnie Shambourger, Former "Mr. Universe"

On the day of the show, I wore an unusual white outfit from Carushka Bodyywear. This outfit really stood out! Even though Ray and I weren't part of the show, of course you all know that I was prancing around meeting everyone. ☺ It's just what I do. Before the show, to my surprise, Yohnnie Shambourger came over to where we were sitting and asked me if I wanted to present trophies to the winners of his show. I was so excited and of course I said yes. He told me he thought I was a body builder but of course I wasn't. After I helped give the winners their trophies, I got the bug of wanting to appear on stage myself. Yohnnie used to do such beautiful body building shows and I wanted to go to all of them. Any time I had a chance to give out those trophies, I wanted to do it.

One day we went out of town to a body building show and I spotted Yohnnie in the audience. Ray pressed me to go talk to Yohnnie about becoming a body builder. I was nervous and didn't want to go talk to him, but I did. Yohnnie told me that he thought I was already a body builder but he said he would work with me.

The next week we talked and he said he would do online training first. He asked me to send him pictures of me in a bathing suit. He then told me how to pose for the pictures and Ray took them and sent them on to Yohnnie. Yohnnie, in turn, sent me a workout program and I was then back to working out with Ray again. He made certain that I followed everything that Yohnnie told me to do, and each month we sent pictures to him of my progress. I really appreciate Ray for all he did for me to keep me focused, and kept me on track. He has always had my best interests at heart and made sure when it was time for me to go to my next level, that he introduced me to the right people to make that happen. I am humbled and honored to call him a dear friend. It is because of him helping me with Yohnie's workout program that I was able to really become the bodybuilder I wanted to be.

When Yohnnie saw I wasn't fooling and saw the changes in my body, he told me he wanted me to come to his center 2 days per week. When I arrived he asked me the following question that I have never forgotten. He asked: "We are about to go on a long journey. Are you ready for it?" I told him that I was. I then told him my story and about fulfilling my sisters dream. I mentioned to him that my thighs had always been a problem for me, but Yohnnie told me not to worry, and with his help, I wouldn't have to worry about them anymore. I had a feeling in my spirit that the real work of fulfilling my sisters vision had only just begun. However, I had made a promise to my sister that I would indeed fulfill her dream and I was determined to do it.

$\mathcal{C}$hapter 6
Taking My Body
To The Next Level

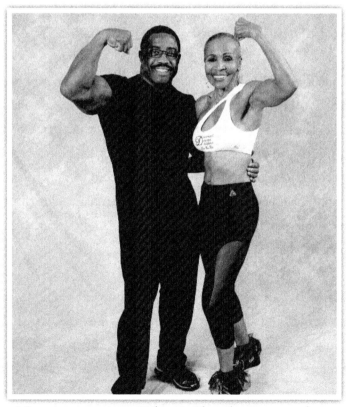

My current trainer, Yohnnie Shambourger, and me.
Photo credit: Maynard Manzano – Magic Glamour Photography

WHEN I STARTED WORKING OUT WITH Yohnnie Shambourger it was a whole new ball game. He never let up on me and I didn't like it sometimes. When I was tired and thought I couldn't do anymore, I would say, "You know I'm old and I love you so much, but I can't do anymore." He would always tell me that he knows but he thought I wanted to fulfill my sisters dream, and if I really wanted to fulfill her dream I had to keep moving. However, he would then jokingly say, "So you are old, and I love you too so keep on doing what I ask." Yohnnie was tough, but that was what I needed to reach my fitness goals.

One of the ladies that I trained at the gym for a short while was Cynthia Evans. She was like a daughter to me and would take time out of her busy schedule to take me back and forth to Washington to train with Yohnnie. That was a lot of wear and tear on her, but she did it without complaint and I appreciate her so very much. When Cynthia couldn't take me, Ernestine Boyd would. I also appreciate Ernestine stepping in when Cynthia was unavailable to take me.

Many days after working out with Yohnnie, I would leave his center and be so tired when I got into the car, all I could do was sleep. I'm so thankful that either Cynthia or Ernestine was driving because there is no way I could have driven home. Yohnnie really worked me hard. I mention this because I don't want anyone to think that it was easy getting my body into shape or that I had an easy road to getting fit and was able to squeak by. No way! It doesn't work like that. It was and still is dedication and hard work to get fit and get your body into shape, especially for a body building show.

After 7 months of extensive training, Yohnnie told me I was ready to compete. I didn't know how to pose, but he taught me. I didn't know where to get my posing outfit, he told Cynthia, and the three of us went to choose a nice suit for me to wear. He told me to choose a good song so I chose "More, More, More – How Do You Like It." We had everything together and now I was ready to do my first body building show.

The day before the show, Cynthia drove me to Washington, helped me check in the hotel and stayed with me. The next day was showtime and I was so nervous. I weighed in at 116 lbs. My pre-judging suit was red velvet. I looked at all the beautiful women and their perfectly toned bodies and I got even more nervous. The one thing I really liked was that the ladies were all very kind to each other. If one needed a pair of earrings from someone and they had an extra pair, they all shared. No one was jealous of the other and that really made me feel more comfortable.

The show started and I was behind the curtain watching the ladies go on stage. They all looked beautiful and the show was going great. Then fear gripped me. All kinds of thoughts were going through my head. Could I do this? Was I good enough? All the modeling I had done and I was never nervous, but this time was different. The difference was I was now outside my comfort zone, and had never done anything like this before. I was really starting to doubt myself. Suddenly, my posing music started to play and it was time for me to walk out on stage. I froze. I started thinking about what my husband might say about the way I was dressed and about my routine. I had failed to mention to him about what I would be wearing. Uh oh! I peeped out the curtain and saw him out there smiling with his hands folded. I stood behind the curtain a few minutes longer and I heard a little voice say, "Ernie, get out there." So I took a deep breath, said a quick prayer and started breathing through the fear. When you get in stressful situations, you have to breathe through the fear and breathe through the little voices in your head and take that step of faith and just go for it.

I went on stage and forgot all about being nervous. I started to have fun and started showing off. Guess what? I didn't want to leave the stage because I was having so much fun. I wished Velvet could have been there and wondered if she was pleased. Deep down I knew that she was.

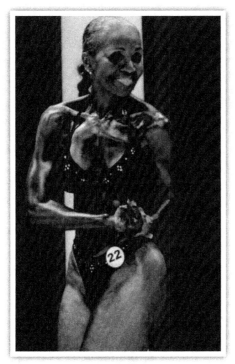

Check out my bicep pose!

After all the women had posed, it was time for the announcement of the winners. As I'm sure you probably guessed, I won in two categories and took home two trophies!

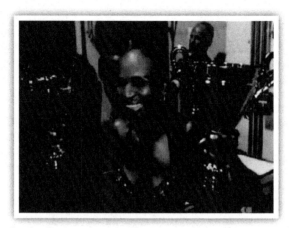

Check out my two trophies I won! I was so excited!

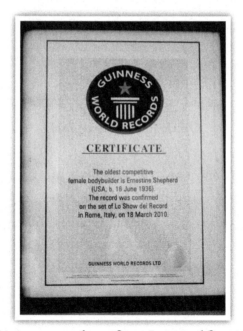

**This is my actual certificate I received from the
Guinness Book of World Records recognizing me
as the Oldest Competitive Female Body Builder
in the world on March 18, 2010.**

In a matter of weeks, Yohnnie got a call from Guinness Book of World Records stating that they thought I was the oldest female body builder in the world, but they would have to check to make sure. It turns out that I was and I was told that I needed to travel to Rome to get my certificate and medal. How exciting and wonderful! I cried tears of happiness because I was finally doing what my sister had wanted.

The night before leaving for Rome, my sister Dee called me crying and told me Velvet had visited her in a dream and told her to write this note to me:

"Teeny, we have accomplished what we wanted. Even in death you did not forget me. I have always been with you but now it is time to set me free. Scatter my ashes in Rome and at any quiet or appropriate moment, please whisper "I set you free, my sister." It is not ironic that you have arrived on my birthday. This is my final gift to you and to us. We have done well but I'm tired now and need to rest. It is now up to you, not anyone else, to set me free. You have held onto me for such a long, long time but it is now time for you to be on your own. At your May show, I will not be there with you. This is your time, not mine, for you have done what you wanted. I have contacted Dee whom we all have listened to since our childhood. She is writing what my voice is telling her to write. Her eyes are closed and I have entered her fingers. Listen to her, I love you and always will, but please set me free for I am tired and need to rest. No longer hold onto my possessions. You have to let me go. I love you very, very much and I will always be in your heart."

I want to let you all in on a secret… to this day, I have NOT let her go. Whenever I am on my speaking engagements, I always carry or wear something of hers. I still buy 2 outfits alike only in different colors. She may be gone, but she will NEVER, EVER be forgotten.

My sisters birthday was March 16 and I arrived in Rome on March 16. The car that picked us up had a tag number of 316. When we arrived at the hotel, the music "You'll Never Walk Alone" was playing and that was Velvet's favorite song. Coincidences? I think not. I could not believe all those things happened to let me know that my sister was there. Her presence was all around us.

However, from that day until this one, good things have come into my life, God has surrounded me with awesome people and the right connections continue to find me.

I also never want to forget that although I loved Velvet very much, God blessed me with two wonderful sisters who have and continue to be in my corner. They are both in good health and doing well, and I thank God for them each and every day. I may not tell my sisters enough, but I sure do love and appreciate them, and I am honored to not only call them my sisters, but also two of my closest friends.

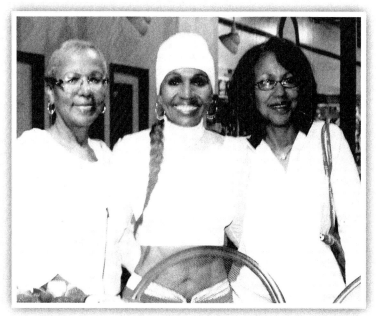

We are family! My sisters Dee, Bern and me.

$\mathscr{C}$hapter 7
The Thorn In My Flesh –
My Battle With Depression

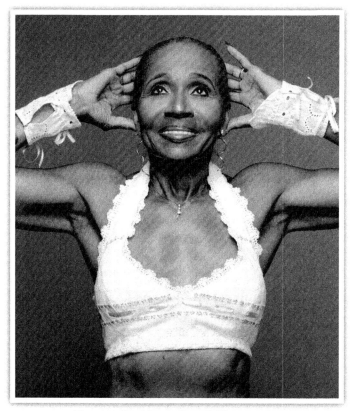

Photo credit: Marvin Joseph Photography

ONE THING I DIDN'T REALLY TALK IN depth about was how I really dealt with my sister's death. I touched on it briefly but wanted to dedicate a chapter to the dark days I had going through the loss of someone I was so close to. This chapter is really my testimony and I am prayerful that it will help someone else going through something similar.

After my sister died, I suffered with deep depression, panic attacks, acid reflux, insomnia, bouts of crying uncontrollably, and I was up walking the floor in the wee hours of the morning. I hated everyone during that time, including myself. I hated God for taking my sister from me and had turned my back on Him. I was a miserable person to be around and I just thank God that my husband and son stuck by me during those really dark, rough days.

One day, while riding the subway, I felt like I wanted to scream and just run up and down the aisle. I have no idea what was wrong with me. A few days later, I went to the hair dresser and while I was waiting for my appointment, I jumped up and ran out of the shop. I jumped in my sons car, which I was driving that day, and I felt like I was closed up in a box. I managed to park the car, called my son and I started screaming on the phone. I told him to come get me because I was just in no condition to drive. He had to leave his car there and take me home in the other car. I got home and went to bed, but I felt like the walls were closing in on me. Emotionally, I was spiraling out of control.

I awakened one morning and felt strange. I can't describe the feeling, all I know is it felt like I had a third arm... yes, a third arm. I looked down and there it was right in the middle of my other arms. I know I was only supposed to have two of them, but there it was. I saw that third arm for awhile and I was very uncomfortable seeing it. I do not know to this day how I dressed and went to work. When I arrived at work the first day I saw it, I told Bern about this other arm. My baby sister, Bern, always knew how to handle me, so she told me all I had to do was hold the third arm or move it out the way. Now I know this may sound weird, but this really happened. I ended up having to work with that third arm for a week. I did not tell my doctor because I thought he would commit me. Even while I was going through that situation, I had the presence of mind to know that the whole thing sounded crazy. After doing extensive research, several medical books referred to what I was going through as "phantom limb" syndrome. This is when a person has a sense that an arm or leg is still attached to the body even after it has been amputated. I was told that I may have associated the third arm with my sister because we were so close to each other. Spiritually and emotionally, it really felt like part of me was cut off when she died.

During that time, I got a lot of support from my husband and my baby sister. Between the two of them I knew I could count on them to help me through it. In addition, as much as I hate taking pills, I unfortunately had to take medicine for my panic attacks, acid reflux, depression and high blood pressure. I also took allergy pills to get drowsy so I could sleep.

My nerves were so bad that my teeth felt like they were loose, my face and fingers tingled and I was in a bad place physically, mentally and emotionally. I could go on and on about all my ailments, that's how bad I was feeling and how low I had sunk in my spirit. I couldn't eat and the times I did, my food stayed in my throat. I really wasn't doing well at all and at the rate I was going, I was on my way to an early grave. I just thank and praise God that Velvet came to me in that dream and told me I was not doing what she asked me to do. This is the thing that straightened me up. Not right away, but that day I made it up in my mind that I was going to fulfill her dream. I knew if I fell completely apart that I would never do what we set out to do. As soon as I got determined to get dedicated and disciplined to be fit, everything changed for me.

My baby sister told me during that time: "Every time you feel like you can't make it, pull out your cute outfit, lace up your tennis shoes and get out and go walking." I decided to listen to her, and I thank Bern for that wonderful advice, because I found that it really worked and still works for me. That is when I decided that I would start walking every day. When I walk, all my worries are gone and all my stress slips away. I pray before I begin my walk and when I return home, I pray again. This one simple addition of walking every day has helped fight my panic attacks and the other illnesses I had without being on any medication. In addition, working hard and following my sisters dream in the gym also made me very happy and kept me grounded and focused.

I know the biggest thing that got me through this rough time in my life was loving God and praising him. Doing this has changed my life completely. I know for a long time I was angry with God and I wasn't His friend anymore. He was always my friend and He always loved me unconditionally, I just stopped talking to Him when Velvet died. I thank Him for forgiving me for being so terrible during that time and His grace and mercy has carried me through that storm and many others in my life. I have learned to just wait on the Lord and wait for His timing. My mother always used to say: "If you wait on the Lord and learn your lessons well, in His timing He will tell you what to do, where to go and what to say, and ultimately everything will work out." My mother was right and I make sure I pray each and every day because I know He brought me out of that deep pit of depression and I thank Him every day for all He has done in my life. To God be the glory!

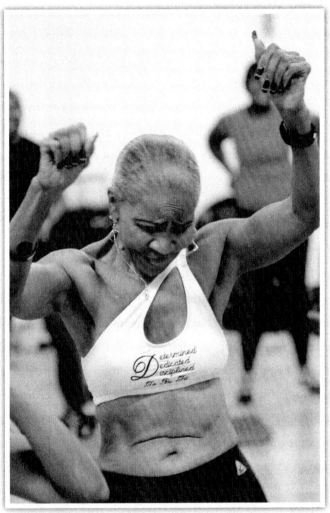

**I am so thankful to God for all He has done in my life.
I just have to give him praise today and every day!**
Photo Credit: Maynard Manzano – Magic Glamour Photography

*C*hapter 8
My Accomplishments

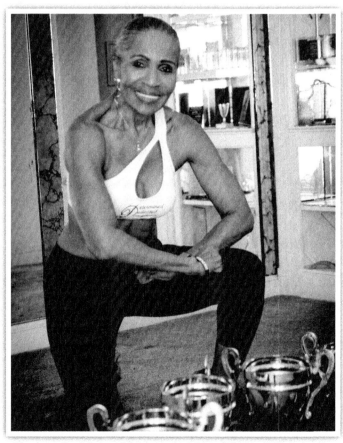

Photo credit: Maynard Manzano – Magic Glamour Photography

OVER THE YEARS, GOD HAS BLESSED ME to receive many accolades and awards of recognition. Although the reason I do what I do is to help others to lead a healthy lifestyle, I am humbled and honored to be recognized. Some of the awards I have received are as follows:

2016 – Howard L. Cornish Humanitarian Award

2015 – Entrepreneurs and Professional Network Legacy Health & Wellness Award

2014 – Muscle Mania Capital Open Womens – 2nd Place

2014 – Masters Womens 60 and over Competition – 3rd Place

2013 – Masters Womens 60 and over Competition – 2nd Place

2013 – Muscle Mania Capital Open Womens – 2nd Place

2012 – Masters Womens 60 and over Competition Grand Master – 1st Place

2011 – Masters Womens 60 and over Competition Grand Master – 1st Place

2010– Guinness Book of World Records Oldest Competitive Female Body Builder In The World

2010– Muscle Mania Capital Open Women's - 2nd Place

2008 – Kina El Yassi NPC Natural East Coast Tournament of Champions Womens 45+ Masters (1st Place)

2008 – Kina El Yassi NPC Natural East Coast Tournament of Champions Womens 45+ Masters (3rd Place)

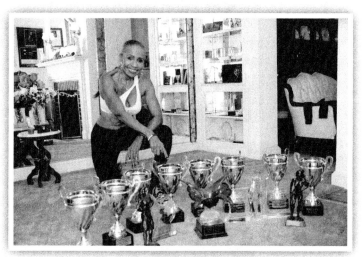

Check out the wonderful trophies and awards I have received. I am humbled and honored.
Photo Credit: Maynard Manzano – Magic Glamour Photography

I have also received numerous medals and certificates of achievement that are too many to list, but I am humbled that so many have taken the time to honor me. Check out my pictures below of my trophies and medals.

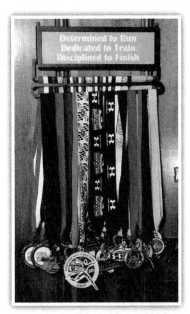

These are a few medals that I have been blessed to receive.
Photo Credit: Maynard Manzano – Magic Glamour Photography

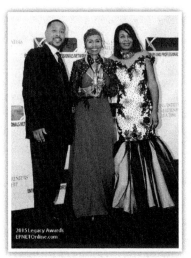

**I was proud to receive the Legacy Health and Wellness
Award on November 14, 2015 from the Founders of
Entrepreneurs and Professionals Network (EPNET). I'm
pictured here with Charles and Theresa Brown, the founders.**

$\mathcal{C}$hapter 9
My Favorite Exercise…
Walking

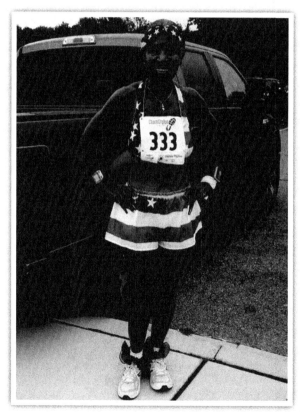

Check out my patriotic colors as I am dressed in red, white and blue, preparing for my 4th of July community walk.

Photo credit: Ernestine Shepherd

My sister Bern was the reason Velvet and I started walking. We found that it was so much fun and we walked around the lake at Hanlon Park. We even dressed up for that. Everything we had on was always matching. My sister could walk very fast and I of course could not. However, I still had fun because we were dressed alike and since the lake was a circle, my sister would pass first and then I would come behind her. People thought I was her and I would laugh and tell them I was just that fast!

When Christmas would come, we would always buy new jackets, hats, gloves and pants. We had so many outfits. After Velvet died I actually stopped walking for awhile. I completely shut down and couldn't bring myself to walk the same paths that she and I had walked. It brought back so many memories and made me sad. However, when I got myself back on track I started walking once again.

When I got back into walking, I met many wonderful people who came out every morning. One lady I met loved to walk and could really walk fast. I called her "Fast Walker." She never missed coming out, and even if it rained she would still be there. One day she told me that she was going to do a marathon. I didn't even know what that was. She did her marathon and got a medal and I teased her and told her I was going to take that medal from her. Then I got to thinking, maybe I could do a marathon but I knew I had to train for it. So I stopped walking around the lake and started walking every morning up Liberty Heights to Liberty Road. I would walk 10 miles out and 10 miles back on Saturday mornings and I knew all the bus drivers that drove the route. At that time I would carry a stick and listen to music on my IPOD. Finally when it was time to sign up for the marathon, I knew I was ready. That cool morning, my husband drove me downtown to walk my first marathon.

When it was almost time to start the walk, my husband was upset and said, "Teeny, I can't leave you. I am afraid something will happen to you." I told him I would be alright but he still didn't want to leave me. There was a young man nearby who overheard us and he said, "Mr. Shepherd, don't worry, I will walk with Ms. Teeny and see that she will be safe." His name was Rob Samson and he did just that. He didn't leave me and stayed with me through the whole marathon. From that time, we became friends and he also became friends with my family. After that, for the next 4 marathons, we were always together. On my 5th marathon, Rob had to go out of town and didn't make it there. I am sure we will do another marathon soon.

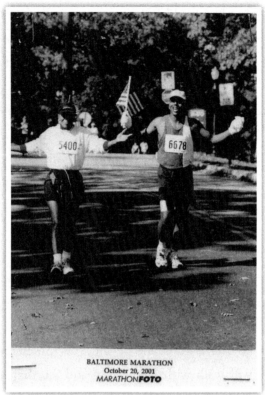

BALTIMORE MARATHON
October 20, 2001
MARATHON**FOTO**

**Picture of Rob Samson and me walking
at my very first Marathon in 2001.**

After the first marathon, I stopped walking up Liberty Road and started walking in Druid Hill Park with my friend Pat Barber. She took me up in the dreaded hills of Druid Hill Park. Although I had never climbed any hills before, I loved it and it made my legs stronger. One day while walking, I met a man named Willie Fitzgerald, who was a runner. I asked him if he thought I could become a runner.

He said, "If you can walk, you can run." He told me he would help me and he did just that. With his help, I started doing 5K's – 10K's, and ½ marathons. He was a very good trainer. We would meet at the park every morning about 5 am before I went to work. At this time I was working at City Springs School, and I never missed a morning training at the park. When I would do my races, Willie was always there with me. Of course you know I introduced him to my family. While Willie and I were running in the park, other ladies joined our group. We had so much fun. All of these ladies were much younger than me and some called me "Ma Ernie."

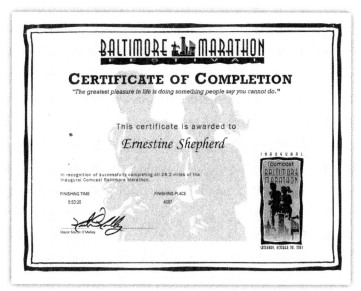

I am so proud of this certificate I received when I completed my very first Marathon! To God be the glory!

It was a cool, late summer morning, and I was on the return loop of my normal 8-12 mile power walk. This is a scenic loop where I encounter many curious on-lookers every day. Sometimes when I'm recognized, I will hear a "Hi Miss Ernestine" or a honk of a horn. On this particular day, I had no idea I was going to encounter a young man that would end up being such a blessing in my life. As I walked, I felt someone walking behind me. As the person walked by, I noticed it was a young man. He smiled and said, "Good morning."

A short while later, I caught up to him and he said, "Hello again, how far are you walking?" I chuckled and replied, "How far are you walking young man?" At this point, he pushed his chest out and said, "Ma'am, you're probably not walking as far as I'm walking, I have about five more miles to go." I smiled and told him the area I was walking to and he then apologized for assuming that I couldn't be walking as far as he was. We both had a good laugh about that. During the next five miles we talked, laughed and spoke about fitness. Since that day I affectionately refer to him as my "fitness son." His name is Chauncey Whitehead.

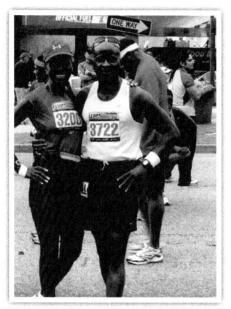

My community walking partner and my "fitness son", Chauncey Whitehead and me.

Through the years, Chauncey and I have participated in numerous fitness and community related events. I also credit my fitness son for training me to run my fastest marathon. A few years had passed and I was struggling with a foot injury that made it difficult for me to run, especially long distances, and the marathon season was approaching fast. Only a few close friends were aware of my injury and I told them I was not physically prepared to run that year.

A few days before the Baltimore running festival, Chauncey informed me he was going to run the half marathon and try to set a personal record (PR). This was significant because all of the previous races he ran with his clients to make sure they crossed the finish line. The morning of the race he saw me and his eyes got bigger than a plate and he said, "Ma what are you doing with a runner's Bib number on?" I replied, "Mama's gonna see what these old legs can do." He looked at me and could tell I was a little apprehensive about running the 13.1 mile distance. Without hesitation he said, "Mama I'm running with you!" I looked at him and said, "Baby you are running your PR today so don't worry about me." He then replied, "It's not about what I can do, it's about helping others!" We ended up running together and whenever I would get tired, had to run up a hill or my injury would start nagging me, he would dial my cell phone so I could hear my ROCKY ringtone. After I heard that ringtone, I would dig deep and keep pressing forward no matter how tired or achy I was feeling. Chauncey and I crossed the finish line together again on that day, and I appreciate him putting his own goals on hold to be there for his "mom". He is a good fitness son.

After I started my community health walk in July, 2013, Chauncey has partnered with me to host these walks on a monthly basis. This community health walk is for all ages and fitness levels, and I'm just so happy that something I started as a way to give back, has taken off and so many are being blessed. If you are in the Baltimore area, feel free to join us. We usually post our schedule on Facebook. I hope to see you at the walk soon. Doing my monthly community walks brings so much joy to me, as well as so many others.

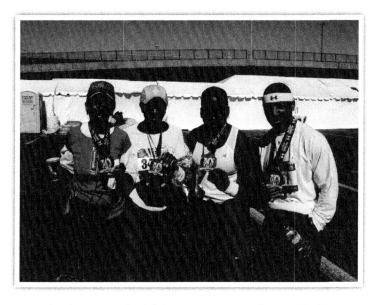

Check out my faithful community walkers, (Thelma Brookes, Chauncey Whitehead, Raymond Day and me).

$\mathcal{C}$hapter 10
Building Muscle and Exercises To Keep Your Body Tight

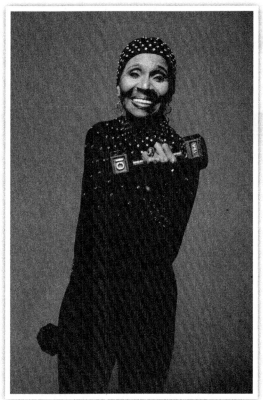

Photo credit: Marvin Joseph Photography

I AM ASKED ON A DAILY BASIS the following question: "What exercises do you do to stay fit?" Well, I have some good news for you! I have decided to give you my top 20 favorite exercises that I do just about every day with my clients, or in my training classes. I divided them by body parts for a total body workout experience. Many of the exercises are done with dumbbells, which will give you a better workout for your body. However, please make sure you use a weight that is manageable for you. If you experience any pain – stop! The movement might be too advanced for you, and you will have to work up to that level. Are you ready to get started? Let's go…

Chest

Combined dumbbell press and dumbbell fly

Lie down on your back with knees bent. *1st part of the combined movement:* Raise the dumbbells above your chest. This will be your starting position. With palms facing outwards, slowly and in a controlled movement, lower the dumbbells down until the upper arms are almost touching the floor. Pause, then raise the dumbbells back up to the starting position. *2nd part of the combined movement:* Turn palms facing each other and lower the dumbbells outwards keeping your elbows slightly bent, slowly and in a controlled movement, lower the dumbbells down until the upper arms are almost touching the floor. Pause, then raise the dumbbells back up to the starting position. Focus on squeezing the chest in order to bring the dumbbells back together. Do 2 sets of 15 reps.

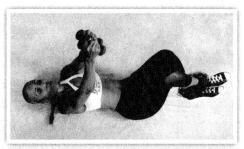

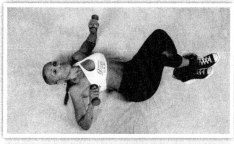

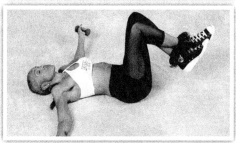

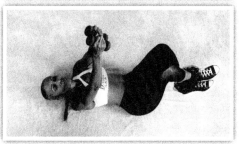

Combined dumbbell fly and thigh adductor

Lie down on your back with legs together, knees slightly bent and holding dumbbell together. Your palms should be facing outward behind your legs. This will be your starting position. Next, lower the dumbbells outwards keeping your elbows slightly bent. Then slowly, and in a controlled movement, open your legs apart simultaneously until the upper arms are almost touching the floor. Pause, then return back to the starting position. Do 2 sets of 15 reps.

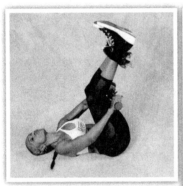
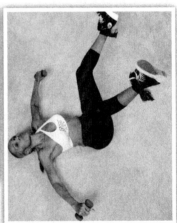
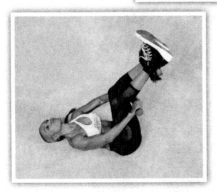

Biceps

Standing dumbbell curl

Stand holding a dumbbell in each hand, with your palms facing outwards. With your elbows to your sides, raise the dumbbell simultaneously until your forearms assume a vertical position. Lower the dumbbells and again maintain the path and the tempo. Do 2 sets of 15 reps.

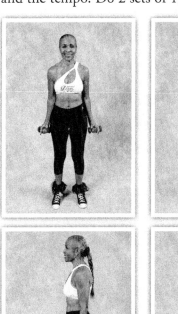
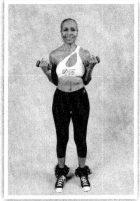
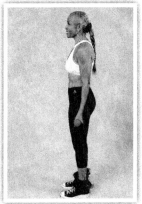
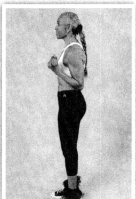

Standing bicep curl

Stand with both arms extended holding a dumbbell in each hand with palms facing upward. This will be your starting position. Simultaneously curl the dumbbell inward until your biceps fully contract. Pause, then return back to the starting position. Do 2 sets of 15 reps.

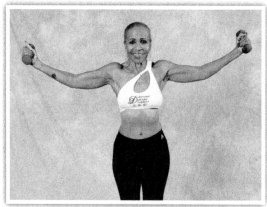

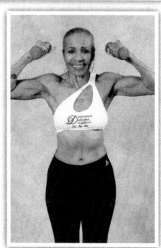

Triceps

Dumbbell kickback

While holding a dumbbell in each hand and palms facing each other, lean your torso forward while your legs are in a straddle position. Now, extend the dumbbells backward with the support of the triceps, while maintaining a stationary position with the other parts of the body. Pause, then return back to the starting position. Do 2 sets of 15 reps.

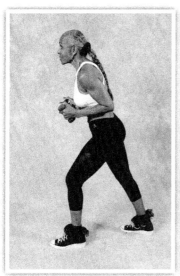
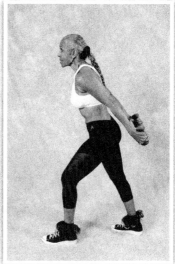

Pushup

Lie on your stomach and place your hands on the floor, slightly wider than a shoulder-width apart. Your feet should be closer than a shoulder-width apart. Push the entire body upward in one movement then lower down without touching the floor again. Do 2 sets of 15 reps.

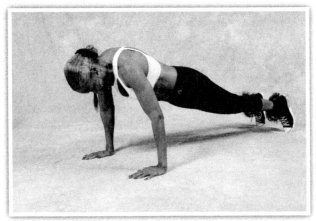

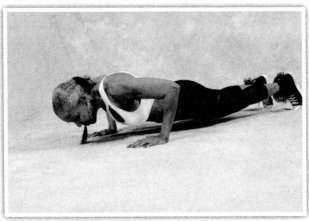

Abdominal and Core

Side T-Plank

Lie on your side with your legs straight and your body in a straight line (shoulders and hips stacked one on top of the other; don't lean forward or backwards). Prop your body up so your hips are off the floor and extend your free arm. Rest your weight on the elbow that's touching the floor. Only your forearm and feet should touch the floor. Do not let the hips sag. Hold for 30 seconds or more.

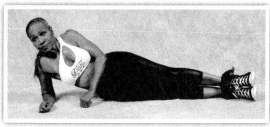

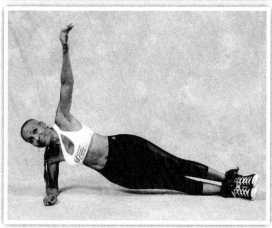

Low Plank

Lie face down on the floor resting on the forearms, with palms flat on the floor. Push off the floor, raising up onto toes and resting on the elbows. Keep body in a straight line from head to toes with no sagging or bending. Hold for 30 seconds or more.

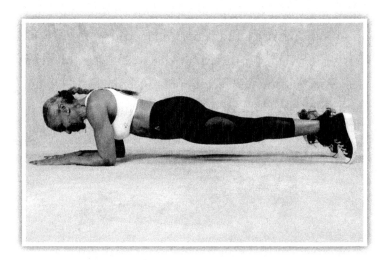

Row-Row-Row Your Boat

Starting from a sitting position on the floor with your knees bent and your heels on the floor. Sit half way up, starting a rowing movement with your arms and upper body. Do 2 sets of 25 reps.

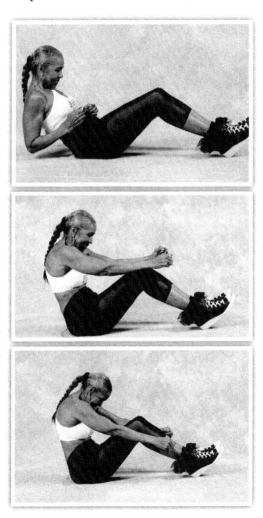

Crunch

A crunch begins with lying face up on the floor with knees bent. The movement begins by curling the shoulders towards the pelvis without tucking your chin into your chest. The hands can be behind or beside the neck. Do 2 sets of 25 reps.

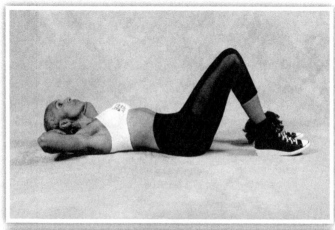

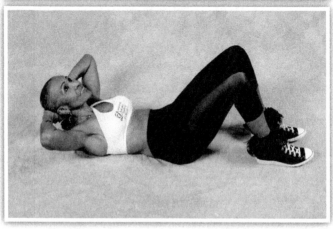

Inverted Bicycle

Lie on your back and roll your hips up into shoulders. This is your starting position. Make sure that you are not too far up on your neck. Your weight should be supported by a nice tripod of your shoulders and upper arms. Then start paddling your legs in a bicycle like motion. Do 2 sets of 25 reps.

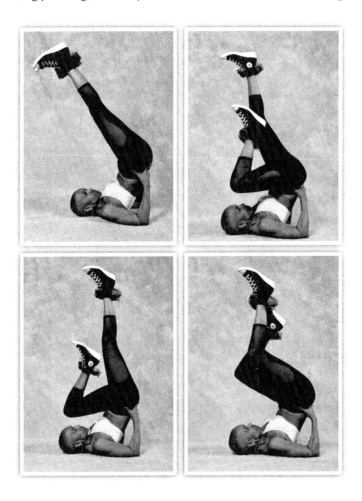

Shoulders

Dumbbell Press

While standing, bend your elbows and raise your upper arms to shoulder height so the dumbbells are at ear level. Push the dumbbells up and in until the ends of the dumbbells are close together, directly over your head, and then lower the dumbbells back to ear level. Do 2 sets of 15 reps.

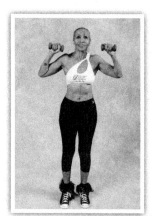
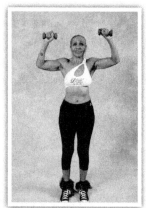
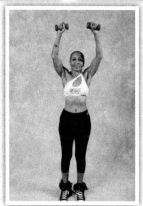

Dumbbell Raise

Stand and hold a dumbbell with each hand at your hips, palms facing each other. Raise the dumbbells to your sides until your arms are at shoulder level and lower them back down after a short pause. Do 2 sets of 10 reps.

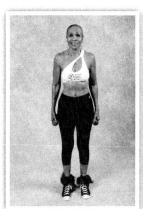
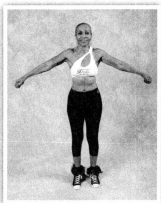
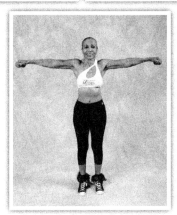

Back

Dumbbell Row

With a dumbbell in each hand, bend forward holding the dumbbells perpendicularly to the floor. Start lifting the dumbbells maintaining close contact between the elbow and the body. Do 2 sets of 15 reps.

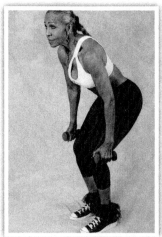 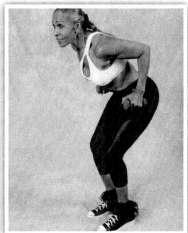

Single Dumbbell Row

Position your legs in a staggered stance. Start with your left arm hanging straight from your shoulder. Keep your back straight and slowly pull the dumbbell up to the side of your rib cage. Then return to the starting position and repeat. Complete the set and repeat with your opposite arm. Do 2 sets of 15 reps.

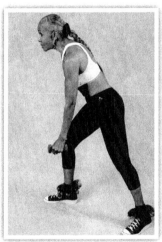
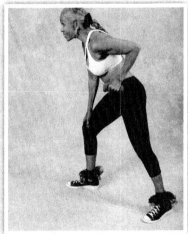

Legs

Plie' Dumbbell Squats

Stand up straight, holding a dumbbell weight that you are comfortable with. Position your feet wider than your shoulders, toes pointed outwards, and start squatting keeping your head up. Do 2 sets of 15 reps.

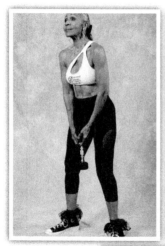
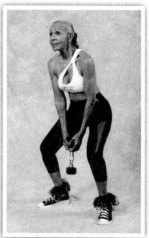
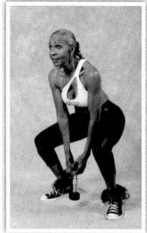

Dumbbell Deadlift

Starting upright, hold dumbbells in each hand. Place your feet shoulder-width apart with the knees slightly bent. This is your starting position. Start lowering the dumbbells while slowly moving in a forward motion, as if you were touching your toes. Lower slightly below your knees then return to starting position. Do 2 sets of 15 reps.

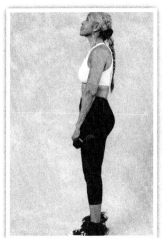 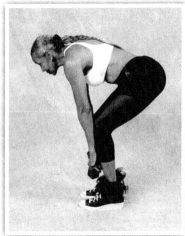

Lying Abductor

Lie down on your right side with your feet stacked together on the floor. Your right hand should be behind your head so that your upper arm lays flat on the ground. Rest your head on your right arm. Begin the exercise by raising your left leg up without bending the leg at all. Raise as high as possible, pause, and then lower back down. Do the movement several times then repeat on opposite side Do 2 sets of 15 reps.

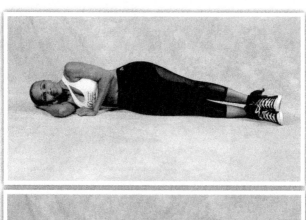

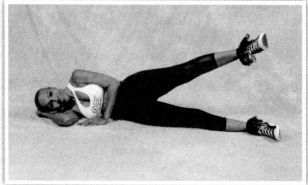

Kneeling Donkey Kickback

Get on your hands and knees. Ensure your back is flat. Be sure to keep your hands on the floor and have them extended out in front of you. Kick the working leg straight back and up. You can make this exercise more effective by contracting the glute muscle when your leg is fully extended. Repeat the movement several times and repeat on the opposite leg. Do 2 sets of 15 reps.

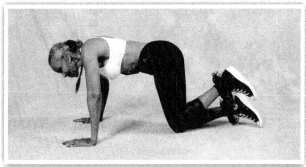

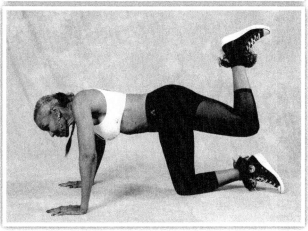

Fire Hydrant

Get on your hands and knees. Ensure your back is flat. Lift your right leg up to the side keeping the knee bent to engage your glute muscle. Repeat the movement several times and repeat on the opposite leg. Do 2 sets of 15 reps.

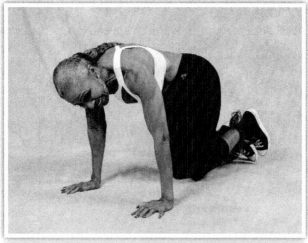

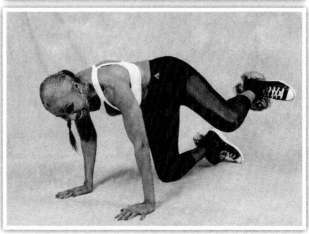

Hip Shaking

Standing with your feet wider than shoulders with arms extended from your side, shake your hips from side to side. Make sure you are having fun. Enjoy dipping and swirling your hips through the movement. Do 2 sets of 45 sec.

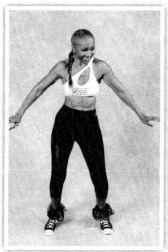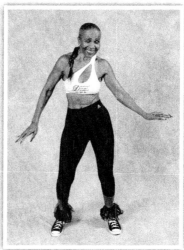

I am confident if you start doing the exercises in this chapter, you WILL get your body in great shape. I also believe that you must practice the 3 D's each and every day. What are the 3 D's? Just in case you didn't know, the 3 D's are:

Determined
Dedicated
Disciplined

$\mathscr{C}$hapter 11
What Can You Eat? Nutrition Tips to Get You Fit!

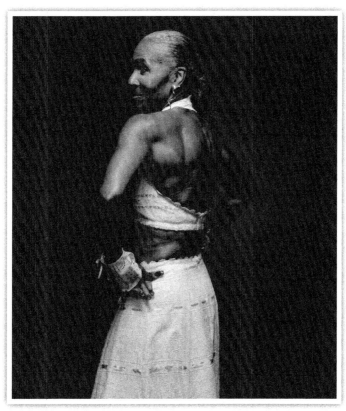

Photo credit: Marvin Joseph Photography

My clients ask me how they should eat to lose weight. I always say that I am not a nutritionist and they should consult one. However, I can tell you about eating clean. Here are a few steps I will share with you. You do not have to be a body builder, runner, or race walker to follow this.

1. Always drink water.

    Why? Your body is made up of about 60% water. Drinking water increases the bodily functions of digestion, absorption, circulation, creation of saliva, transportation of nutrients, and maintenance of body temperature. It will also flush the body of junk you have been eating.

2. Get rid of all the junk food in your house and replace with food choices like lean red meat, chicken, eggs, tuna, fish (tilapia, cod, salmon, haddock, trout), yams and white potatoes. Watch your bread intake because those carbohydrates can easily cause you to gain weight.

3. Create a daily food journal writing down everything you eat and drink. Keeping a journal is like seeing a day's worth of food laid out in front of you. You can immediately identify your good and bad habits, and this helps keep you accountable. You can find a free food journal online or download an app to your smart

phone. I prefer to make my own using a notebook. Include: Day, Meal (breakfast, snack, lunch, etc.), time of meal, serving size, amount of water, and review of day.

4. You can't do this alone. Always pray each day about eating healthy and if you do this, your prayers will be answered. It took awhile but it worked for me.

5. Get in at least 45 minutes of any type of cardio that you like to do. Doing this will ensure you will do it daily. I do cardio 6 days a week. But if you are a beginner, try 15 minutes three days a week until you can do more. I started with 15 minutes of non-stop dancing three days a week at home, and I enjoyed every minute of it!

6. Last but not least, preparation is the key to everything. Take the time to prepare your meals for the week and you will have a greater chance for success.

SPECIAL NOTE: Before trying my diet ask your doctor about taking extra protein and what kind. Remember, my meal plan works for my body, but it may not be the best meal plan for **YOU!**

Meal 1

1 cup oatmeal (quick or whole oats)

½ cup Pineapple-canned in its own juice

1 tbs chopped English Walnuts

8 oz glass of liquid egg whites = 26g of protein

Meal 2

4 oz. can tuna packed in water

1 cup Spinach -leaf frozen all natural no preservatives

3 oz sweet potato -baked in skin

8 oz glass of liquid egg whites

Meal 3

3 oz Turkey white meat roasted

1 cup green beans frozen -cooked

1 cup brown rice – cooked

Meal 4

4 oz chicken breast no skin baked

1 cup broccoli cooked from frozen

3 oz sweet potato

8 oz glass of liquid egg whites

Meal 5

4 oz can of tuna (same as above)

1 cup Asparagus

8 oz glass of liquid egg whites

After working out at the gym, I drink an 8oz glass of liquid egg whites, and an 8oz glass before going to bed. I also drink 16oz of water after each meal.

I hope my nutrition suggestions will help you reach your own personal goals, and guide you on your journey to get Determined, Dedicated and Disciplined to be fit!

$\mathcal{C}$hapter 12
Motivational Quotes To Get You Determined, Dedicated and Disciplined

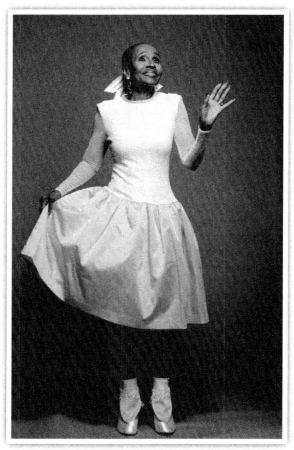

Photo credit: Marvin Joseph Photography

EVERY DAY WHEN I GET UP, I say my devotions, pray and say daily affirmations and motivation to get me going each day. Below are daily devotions and words of encouragement that I read each day and say each day and I invite you to do the same.

Daily Devotions:

Dear God,

I give this day to You.

May my mind stay centered on the things of spirit.

May I not be tempted to stray from love.

As I begin this day, I open to receive You.

Please enter where You already abide.

May my mind and heart be pure and true, and may I not deviate from the things of goodness.

May I see the love and innocence in all mankind,

behind the masks we all wear and the illusions of this worldly plane.

I surrender to You my doings this day.

I ask only that they serve You and the healing of the world.

May I bring Your love and goodness with me, to give unto others wherever I go.

Make me the person You would have me be.

Direct my footsteps, and show me what You would have me do.

Make the world a safer, more beautiful place.

Bless all Your creatures.

Heal us all, and use me, dear Lord, that I might know the joy of being used by You. Amen.

(Excerpted from ILLUMINATA by Marianne Williamson)

Motivational Quotes That Keep Me Inspired:

"Always be Determined, Dedicated and Disciplined in whatever you do." *(Ernestine Shepherd)*

"Age is nothing but a number, and you can get fit." *(Ernestine Shepherd)*

"If ever there were an anti-aging pill, it would have to be exercise." *(Ernestine Shepherd)*

"Whatever you do, do with kindness. Whatever you say, say with kindness. Where ever you go, radiate kindness." *(Unknown)*

"What is age but a number. What you can dream, you can become at any age. Live your best life not your age." *(Unknown)*

"You are never too old to set another goal or to dream a new dream." *(Unknown)*

"Spread love everywhere you go. Let no one come to you without leaving happier." *(Mother Teresa)*

"Our happiness depends on the habit of mind we cultivate. So practice happy thinking every day. Cultivate the merry heart, develop the happiness habit, and life will become a continual feast." *(Norman Vincent Peale)*

"Be the living expression of God's kindness. Kindness in your face, kindness in your eyes, and kindness in your smile." *(Unknown)*

"To leave the world a better place and to know even one life has breathed easier because you have lived, this is to have succeeded." *(Ralph Waldo Emerson)*

"Tell God your needs and don't forget to thank him. When you do this you will experience God's peace, which is far more wonderful than the human mind can understand. His peace will keep your thoughts, and heart quiet and at rest as you trust in Christ Jesus." *(Unknown)*

"Happiness cannot be found when you seek it for yourself. However, when you give it to others, it will find it's way back to you. That's the mystery of happiness... it grows when shared." *(Unknown)*

"The sum of the whole is this: Walk and be happy, and walk and be healthy. The best way to lengthen out our days is to walk steadily and with a purpose". *(Unknown)*

$\mathcal{C}$hapter 13
Frequently Asked Questions
and Answers From Ernestine

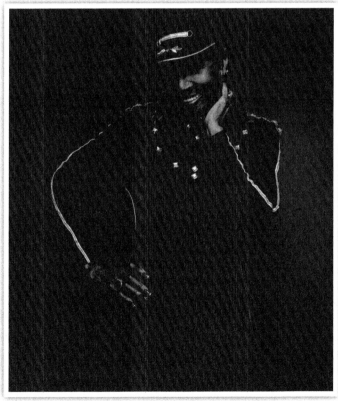

Photo credit: Marvin Joseph Photography

How slow/fast did you ease into working out initially? Short period/every day/every other day? Any recommendations for those just starting out?

I started out doing aerobics two days a week for an hour each time. I did this for 5 months and then I started doing the aerobics for a half hour, and then weight training for a half an hour two days a week. I did this for about a year.

Looking back on your beginning moments, what lessons did you learn and what would you do differently?

I wouldn't have done anything differently. I believe that the path God has put you on is the way things are meant to be. I did learn that when you are working out and going for a goal, you have to be consistent. I also learned you have to have fun in everything you do. Finally, I learned that my age didn't matter. Even though I started later in life working out, I began where I was and made a new ending.

I often have a hard time relating to trainers, who are very young & not super excited to work with wrinkly older ladies. How can I motivate them to push me and get excited about working with me?

Unfortunately, there is no way you can push a person to work out with you. If they don't have the patience or passion to work out with you, then they aren't who you want to work out with anyway. Furthermore, don't call yourself "wrinkly older ladies". Don't carry yourself as being "wrinkly" or "old" and maybe a younger trainer will work out with you.

How did you deal with depression and what role did your fitness journey play in helping you through it? I would also like to know if you had or have days you just don't feel like moving and if so, what do you do?

I dealt with my depression by praying every day and meditation helped as well. I would also get my clothes on and go walk. I found out that a good walk helps. Then I would go to the gym and being around other people made me get out of my depressed mood. It also changed my way of thinking. I find that until this day, I have to keep moving to keep my spirits up and my mind clear. I never have days that I don't feel like moving because I know it is good for me and I enjoy being around people, and love what I do.

Living on the East Coast, I know you have more brutal winters. I'm from California and I'm a wimp when it

comes to the weather. When I come home from work and if it's dark and cold, I will then huddle by the heater, put on my robe, and it's over. I will be in for the evening. Working out goes out the window. Help! How do you stay motivated to keep moving in the winter?

Staying motivated is easy because I enjoy what I do. It is a joy to run/walk. It is very good for me and it keeps my mind clear and it truly helps me stay on task. I also like being around people. My ministry after my sister died, is to help others live a happy, healthy lifestyle, and I must practice what I preach.

Do you have any tips for finding a buddy to exercise with? Or starting a healthy habits meet-up group?

You have to be in a place where people are working out to find a buddy. Going to an actual gym that has a lot of people in it will help. Surround yourself with like-minded people, and you will eventually find someone to buddy up with.

How long will it take for exercise to affect your health, especially blood pressure and cholesterol?

It depends on the individual person. It's not just exercise, it is how you are eating. You must also talk to your doctor to find out what is the best exercise program for your body.

I would like to learn how to train to become stronger. Especially since I believe I will live into my 100's. How do I begin?

What I did was start off slow with the aerobics and then walking. Then I ate healthy and drank plenty of water. This is good for your fitness journey. Be patient and don't rush it, it will come.

What was that one defining moment in your life when you realized "I have to really & truly take care of my body for the long haul as it is a temple of the Holy Spirit who lives in me?"

What made me start was following my sisters dream of inspiring others to live more healthy, happy and productive lives. After suffering with depression, what worked for me was exercise and I knew that I had to make it a daily part of my life in order for me to feel and look my very best.

When you're invited to a lot of events on a regular basis what is the best way to get through them while sticking to your eating plan and without drawing attention to yourself?

I made up my mind that I would be determined to eat healthy and anyone who knows me, knows that is how I am. I'm also not paying attention to people paying attention to what I am eating. I am sticking to what I said I was going to do and that is eating healthy so I practice what I preach.

What made you stay focused and how did you get through the plateaus?

What helped me stay focused was that I started working out with my sister TOGETHER. She was my accountability partner and that kept me on track. We also had a plan and we knew we had to try to help others live a healthy lifestyle.

What do you do, or think about, to motivate you when you have exercised routinely for several months, but then the holidays come around and you can't get yourself back into the gym?

What motivates me is that exercise is the thing that makes me happy. I never take time off for holidays. If you can't go to the gym, you have to find the time to work out in your home. The mistake people make is taking time off for the holidays. Keep working out all the time. There are no work out vacations because even when you are on vacation, you should still work out.

How you would describe your emotional/spiritual disposition since you became fit?

Now that I have become physically fit, I thank God for the strength and courage to keep exercising. Without Him none of this would be possible. When I first started, I wasn't as spiritual as I am now. After I had the tragedy of losing my sister, everything changed. I changed, mentally, spiritually and emotionally, and I'm a better person all the way around.

How often should you work out a week to achieve your goals without damaging ourselves?

I work out 3 days per week (Mon - Wed- Fri) and I have been doing that for the past 24 years. I have a set schedule and keep to it. It hasn't harmed my body in any way. I also walk/run approximately 7 days out of the week, and I feel better now then I did when I was in my forties.

When you decided to get in the best shape of your life how did you change your self-image from what it was before? What changed for you and how do you maintain that new self-image?

What initially made me start working out is that my sister and I didn't like the way we looked in our bathing suits. We made a decision to change our physique so that we felt good about ourselves. After we started working out and seeing results we got more confidence in how we looked and it made our self-esteem soar.

How do you fuel your workouts? Also do you take any supplements?

I don't take any supplements. To fuel my workouts, I drink an 8 ounce glass of liquid egg whites and sometimes I will eat an energy bar after my run/walk.

Have you had to deal with injuries?

From all the walking/running I have done, I developed Plantar Fasciitis in my right foot. I had it for about 6 months. I have always had flat feet and I didn't realize I needed tennis shoes that were motion controlled to keep my feet from going inward and that also provided support. I also had to put custom made orthotic insoles in my shoes. In addition, I went to therapy to help correct the problem.

Have you taken any hormone replacement after menopause? How did you get through it?

I never took any hormone replacement pills and I was blessed to have a relatively symptom free menopause. I didn't have hot flashes or any other female problems. I am grateful to God that He spared me.

Cellulite! You said you had cellulite before you started working out and that your legs were a mess. Please tell me there is hope!

There is hope! You have to change the way you are eating and you have to work the legs and do certain exercises that really target that area. Find one that is not going to be too stressful or injurious to you. Keep the faith, there is hope!

What are your beauty secrets for beautiful skin?

- I don't eat junk food.

- I drink plenty of water.

- I don't lay out in the sun a lot. I do get a little sun but not a lot.

- I don't use straight soap to cleanse my skin, but cleanse with a good skincare regime.

Are you up early to start your routine purposely or you start your routine whatever time you arise?

I am up early on purpose. I get up early to do my devotions, then I eat and then I go out to run/walk.

Why do you get up so early? I'm DYING to know! And what time do you go to bed?

I get up at 2:30 am every morning because my body clock has just gotten used to it. I usually go to bed at different times. Some nights I go to bed at 9 PM, sometimes I go to bed later, it all depends on what is going on.

If you could only choose one fitness activity today - what would it be and why?

The one activity I love is working out my back. I love the pull downs, chin ups, anything dealing with the back. I feel that is the strongest part of my body and I feel that my back is defined very well.

What do you eat when eating out at restaurants and with friends?

I can eat turkey, chicken (baked or grilled), baked potato, sweet potato, brown rice and vegetables with no preservatives.

**What strategies do you use, in overcoming obstacles &
staying determined, dedicated & disciplined?**

I enjoy what I do and I made a promise to my sister 24
years ago that I would continue her dream. Also God is in
my life and He helps me to keep going. Everywhere that I
go and in everything I do God is always there to help me
stay determined, dedicated and disciplined to be fit.

$\mathscr{C}$hapter 14
Fitness Action Plan...
How To Get Started

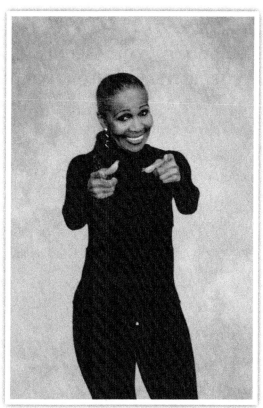

Photo credit: Maynard Manzano – Magic Glamour Photography

My journey is still being written but most of you have this question swirling around in your head: "How do I start my own fitness journey?"

The answer is really simple: **You have to start.**

Please read the words I am about to say and let them sink into your soul and spirit:

You must stop wishing, planning, hoping and watching others get into shape. You have to make up your mind that you are going to **DO IT!** Get **DETERMINED** that you are going to get **DEDICATED** and **DISCIPLINED** to be fit!

Above is the short and simple answer, but for those of you who need some steps to ACTUALLY kick off your own personal action plan, the key steps are:

- Start slow,
- Start moving,
- Start walking,
- Start stretching,
- Start praying,
- Start living,
- Start DOING!

*__Special Note:__ Please consult your doctor before starting any new fitness plan.

I am confident you can do it, and I'm praying for your success. Continue to ask God to lead you and guide you on your journey and you will be well on your way to being fit for life.

Acknowledgements

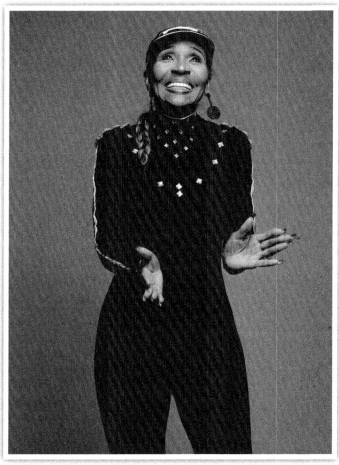

Photo credit: Marvin Joseph Photography

Throughout my book I have mentioned several people who have helped me along the way, but I want to dedicate this section to a few special people who I love, adore and respect:

Family:

My Parents – Milton and Ernestine Hawkins (Deceased)

Thank you to my parents because without you, there would be no me. I think of you both every day and I thank God that you are the parents that raised me. I love you both always.

My Sister Dim/Velvet – Mildred Hawkins (Deceased)

Thank you dear sister for being my closest friend over the years. Even though you may not physically be here, you still live on and your legacy will never die. I know you are looking down from heaven and watching over me every day and I am grateful. I just want you to know that your dream is alive and well, and this book will touch people all over the world. We did it dear sister... we did it! You may be gone but you are never, ever forgotten. I love you forever.

My sister Dee – Eleanora Hawkins Morton

Thank you for challenging me and standing beside me throughout my long journey. You always told me that everything would be alright and offered me a hug at the end of the day when I needed it the most. When I had questions while writing this book, I could always count on you to help me find a solution. Thank you for encouraging me to write this book and I love you dear sister.

My brother Micky – Milton Hawkins

Thank you for your encouragement. You always called me "Baby Teen" and you were always in my corner when we were children. Now you always say to me, "You are strong, follow Dim and follow your dreams." I love you dear brother.

My brother Bobby - Robert Hawkins (Deceased)

Thank you for always having such a joyful spirit and telling me all the time how proud you were of me and Dim. You also always told me to follow my dreams and I am doing just that. I love you always dear brother.

My sister Bunny/Bern – Bernice Hawkins-Whelchel

Thank you for being so tough on me after Dim's death. You made me see that I was strong even when I thought I could not make it through another day. Your "tough love" helped more than you know and I love you very much.

My husband – Collin J. Shepherd and son – Michael Shepherd

Thank you for loving me unconditionally and loving me past my pain. Losing my sister was very hard on me and I know I was pretty tough to take for a long time after her death. I dedicated this book to the two of you because you are indeed the wind beneath my wings. Your love lifted me out of the deep pit of depression and I thank you and love you both very, very much.

My best friend – Ernestine Boyd

Thank you for being my best friend all these years. You have been a constant source of encouragement and my sister from another mother. I appreciate you and love you more than words can say dear friend.

My cousin – Thelma Brookes

Thank you for being part of my work outs and walks in the morning, attending my classes, always supports all my endeavors and just for being there when I need you. I also appreciate you being so instrumental in me receiving the Charles L. Cornish Award earlier this year. Thank you dear cousin. I love you.

My niece (Velvet's Daughter) – Dietra Johnson

Thank you for being part of my life. For 24 years after your mother's death, you call to check on me every morning and every night. No matter what, I know I can count on you and I thank you for just being you. I love you my dear niece.

Pastor William E. Butler

I have been a proud member of Union Memorial United Methodist Church for over 50 years. Thank you to my Pastor and his wife for spiritual guidance and to my entire church family at Union Memorial United Methodist Church, 2500 Harlem Avenue, Baltimore, MD 21215

Extra Special Thank You's:

Jay Bennett

Special thank you to Jay Bennett for being the very first person to take me on this long fitness journey. It has been a long journey but you were the first person to see something in me that I didn't see in myself and I will forever be grateful.

Raymond Day

Special thank you to Ray for being the second person to work with me and taking me to another level on this journey. I also love that when you recognized it was time for me to go to another level, you introduced me to the person who could get my body to the place it needed to be. I appreciate our 24 years of friendship and I don't take it for granted all you have done in my life. You have been my main accountability partner over the years, and have been with me through the thick and thin. I appreciate you so very much my friend.

Yohnnie Shambourger

Special thank you to Yohnnie for all you have done for me on this journey into fitness. Your constant support and help during these last 9 years have been invaluable and I thank you for pushing me into my next level. I also appreciate when Ray introduced us that you took a chance on me and helped me get my body into the best shape of my life.

Betty Fenner-Davis of Fenner Originale

Special thank you to Betty Fenner for being my personal fashion designer and stylist for well over 30 years. You have helped me with my image and style, and have developed all the amazing outfits that I wear to all my functions. When my sister passed, my perspective changed and I found a renewed purpose. All my outfits changed to active wear and I challenged you to create totally new looks for me and, as always, you rose to the challenge. I appreciate all you have done for me, and look forward to what we will do next.

Linda M. Hollis

Special thank you to Linda Hollis for being my friend and Personal Assistant for 3 ½ years. We always have a wonderful time traveling together. You know I am the body builder, but you not only take care of my itinerary, but you also lift my baggage on the plane because I can't do it by myself. ☺ ☺ Often during my speaking engagements, you so graciously demonstrate many of the exercises I teach. I love our routine we have developed during our travels when our hosts invite us to a meal and after we finish they will be completely surprised when I ask you for a cigarette. At that time, being the health and fitness guru that I am, our hosts will look at us with complete disbelief and surprise. Every time you pull out the pack of gum, we always have a good laugh. You are a wonderful friend and assistant and I appreciate you very much.

Mack Hardison

Special thank you to Mack Hardison for still being my friend all these years. We go back to our days working together at Western Electric. Through the years, if I would be singing with the band, doing fashion shows or whatever you would always yell out, "Go Ernie, do it!" A few years ago I traveled to Richmond to do a presentation and I remember you were there because you live out that way. I'll never forget that I wore an outfit with a pink jacket and after I had talked for awhile, I threw my jacket out in the audience and people tried to catch it. Thank God you caught it for me because I wanted it back. ☺ People thought whoever caught it could keep it. I know you had a hard time holding onto my jacket because everyone wanted it. After the event, I appreciate you bringing my jacket to me but I'll also never forget you said, "Ernie, I'm going to get you for that one." I couldn't ask for a better friend over the years and I appreciate you.

Youfit Gym

I want to give an extra special thank you to Youfit Gym in Randallstown, MD for all they have done for me. I have been a trainer there for many years and they have always been so gracious and kind. Whenever I need to have photo shoots or any special requests, they are ready, willing and able to assist. All the staff are very friendly, and the gym is neatly kept. I couldn't ask for a better fitness facility partner, and I look forward to my long-term relationship with Youfit.

Theresa Royal Brown

Finally, an extra special thank you to my newly "adopted" daughter, Theresa Royal Brown. You and your team have worked tirelessly with me to get this book published. Without your faithfulness to this project and your unwavering support, this book would not have been possible. You truly went above and beyond the call of duty on so many levels and I thank God He brought you into my life originally back in 2011 and then again in 2015. The late nights, the countless changes and revisions and your many trips to Baltimore to meet with me, really speaks to your commitment not only to me, but to this project and I appreciate you very much for bringing this book to life. I also appreciate you joining my team as my event planner heading up my national/international book tour. The work has just begun but I thank you for helping to make this happen.

No matter what you do in life, you can never do it alone. All of these wonderful people helped me on my fitness journey in some way, shape or form and I want to take this time to acknowledge them:

Fitness Life

Jay Bennett
Dr. Edna Simmons
Raymond Day
Ernest Jones
Yohnnie Shambourger
Sheritha McKenzie

Nutrition
Todd Swinney

Dave Spindell

Walking
Bernice Whelchel

Pat Barber

Rob Samson

Running
Willie Fitzgerald

Remus Medley

Chauncey Whitehead

3:30 am Runners
Wally Gumbs

Linda Hollis

Wendy Berry

Drena

Ronald Dupye

5:30 am Runners
Willie Fitzgerald

Gail Austin

Thelma Brookes

Wendy Berry

Maysa

Etolie Diggs

Niki Dickerson

Patra Jones

Marathon Runners

Gail Austin

Thelma Brookes

Niki Dickerson

Etolie Diggs

Friends From Western Electric

Edwina Weaver

Mildred Burroughs (Deceased)

Mack Hardison

William Cheatham

Additional Family

All my nieces and nephews

Cousins - Marguerite Smith/Vonzella Jones

Velvet's Grandson - Keith Johnson (Lovie)

My grandson - Michael Wilson

Community Walkers

Faith Bennett

Thelma Brooks

Raymond Day

Chauncey Whitehead

Church Exercise Group

Brenda Brown

Marguerite Smith (Deceased)

Sharon Woods

Jacqueline Anderson

Transportation

Wally Gumbs

Cynthia Evans

Ernestine Boyd

Linda Hollis

Ronald Dupye

Food

Eggs International

Gym

You Fit

Book Project

Theresa Royal Brown

Charles Brown

Keith Burns

Marvin Joseph
Maynard Manzano
Yohnnie Shambourger
Carolyn Sheltraw

God placed all of these beautiful people in my fitness life. Each and every one of them helped me to climb until my sister's dream came true. A poem by Helen Steiner Rice was given to me years ago by Velvet and I want to dedicate it to all of the individuals I just named:

Climb 'Til Your Dream Comes True

Often your tasks will be many,

And more than you think you can do.

Often the road will be rugged

And the hills insurmountable, too.

But always remember, the hills ahead

Are never as steep as they seem,

And with Faith in your heart start upward

And climb 'Til you reach your dream.

For nothing in life that is worthy

Is never too hard to achieve

If you have the courage to try it

And you have the Faith to believe.

For Faith is a force that is greater

Than knowledge or power or skill

And many defeats turn to triumph

If you trust in God's wisdom and will.

For Faith is a mover of mountains.

There's nothing that God cannot do,

So start out today with Faith in your heart

And "Climb 'Til Your Dream Comes True" !

- Helen Steiner Rice (1900 - 1981)

$\mathcal{A}$uthor Highlights

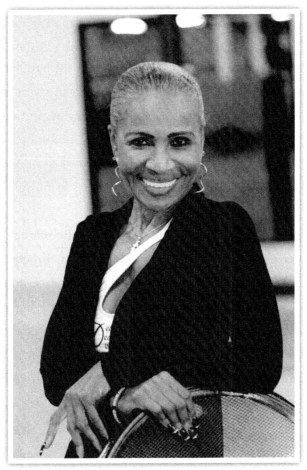

Photo credit: Maynard Manzano - Magic Glamour Photography

Ernestine Shepherd

ERNESTINE SHEPHERD IS A FITNESS GURU in her own right, whose mantra for the past 24 years has been, "Determined, Dedicated - Disciplined To Be Fit For Life." She believes that it is never too late to become physically fit and that "Age Is Nothing But A Number."

At the age of 56, she began working out at Coppin State College with her sister. The story goes that she and her sister were displeased with how they looked in swim suits, and decided to do something about it. They began to train vigorously, but unfortunately, her sister succumbed to a brain aneurysm. However, Ernestine decided to work even harder and vowed to carry on in her sister's memory.

She has been married for 60 years and is the mother of a 59-year old son and a 19-year old grandson. Ernestine is truly an inspiration to all who meet her. Her fashion is above reproach and she is easily recognized by her gray, pushed back hair with her long braid extending down her back. In addition, she is always dressed in her colorful outfits embossed with her mantra, and her decorative high heel tennis shoes.

Two of her favorite songs are, "Here I Am Lord", and "This Little Light of Mine". Her "little light" is her energy and eagerness to take time out of her busy schedule to hold classes for seniors at her church, at various community organizations and particularly at the YouFit Health and Wellness Center in Baltimore. Her favorite Bible verses are I Corinthians, Chapter 13 and the 23rd Psalm. Ernestine strongly believes that it is extremely important for Christians to actively live out their faith

Overall her most inspirational song is "One Moment In Time" by Whitney Houston. To paraphrase the song, Ms. Ernestine says, "Life is a race against destiny, but we are all given that one moment in time to be the best that we can be."

HIGHLIGHTS:

- Television appearances: Oprah, Katie Couric, Anderson Cooper, Roland Martin, CNN, ABC News, Good Morning America, Inside Edition, 700 Club and the Mo'Nique Show

- Currently featured in "Ripley's Believe It Or Not!" book as Granny's Six-Pack

- Featured in Guinness Book of World Records Winner as "Oldest Female Body Builder. Received award in Rome, Italy in March, 2010

- Competed in seven 5K, 10K and marathon runs coming in first place for her age group

- Featured in Prevention Magazine, Essence Magazine, Jet Magazine and Ebony Magazine

Ernestine is on a worldwide mission to spread the message of wellness, fitness and eating right no matter what your age. Her favorite saying is and always will be… "Age Is Nothing But A Number."

$\mathcal{B}$ook Tour Cities
For 2016

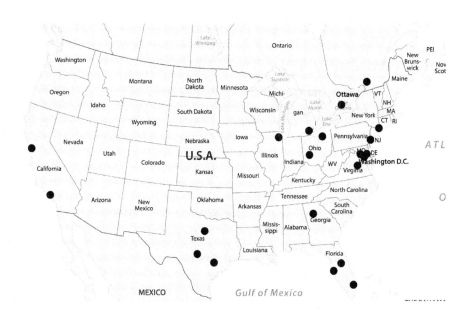

To MARKET MY FIRST BOOK, WE WILL be launching a 3 segment book tour. The first segment will be for the USA only. The second segment will be for Canada and the third segment will be overseas. The dates will be announced shortly and more details on all 3 segments will be sent out via social media, i.e., Facebook, Twitter, Instagram, etc. Be on the look-out and I hope to see you in person!

Book Tour Tentative Segments and Cities:

Segment I – USA
(DMV Area)
Greenbelt, MD
Baltimore, MD
Washington, DC
Richmond, VA
New York, NY
Chicago, IL
Philadelphia, PA
Detroit, MI
Los Angeles, CA
San Francisco, CA
Miami, FL
Orlando, FL
Tampa, FL
Austin, TX

Dallas, TX
Houston, TX
Atlanta, GA
Cincinnati, OH
Cleveland, OH
(Proposed cities subject to change)

Segment II – Canada
Montreal
Ontario
Toronto

Segment III – United Kingdom/Australia/Asia (2017)

*H*ow To Book Ernestine

Ernestine Shepherd is an American bodybuilder, she is probably best known for being, at one point, the oldest competitive female bodybuilder in the world, as declared by the *Guinness Book of World Records* in 2010 and 2011. Ernestine trains others each week as well as continues to work with her personal trainer, Yohnnie Shambourger to stay physically fit.

Ernestine is available for speaking engagements. Please go to: www.ernestineshepherd.net for more information on how she can be part of your event.

Thank You From Ernestine!

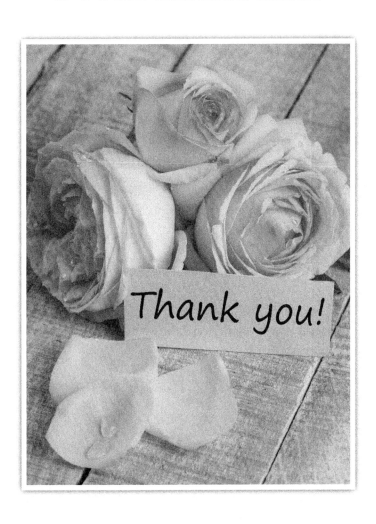

THANK **YOU** FOR PURCHASING A COPY OF this book and taking a sneak peak into my life.

I hope this book was a blessing to you and that you learned a lot more about me and my journey. I also hope that something that I said motivated you and inspired you to get determined to be fit.

Please let me hear from you! I invite you to send me a testimonial and any feedback about the book to: **info@agelessjourneybook.com**

As you may have heard, my team and I are also working on an upcoming retreat where I will be working up close and personal with those of you who are ready to step outside your comfort zone and spend a couple of days with me to get fit. If you are interested in being part of the retreat, send an email to **info@agelessjourneybook.com**. In the subject line type in: **"Send Retreat Info"** and we will send you the detailed email on how you can sign up. We can only accept 100 people, therefore, if you want to attend, make a decision to be there and sign up early.

Finally, if you would like to purchase additional copies of this book, go to:
www.agelessjourneybook.com

Stay focused on your goals, always remember that age is nothing but a number and stay Determined, Dedicated and Disciplined to be fit!

I love you and God bless!

Ernestine

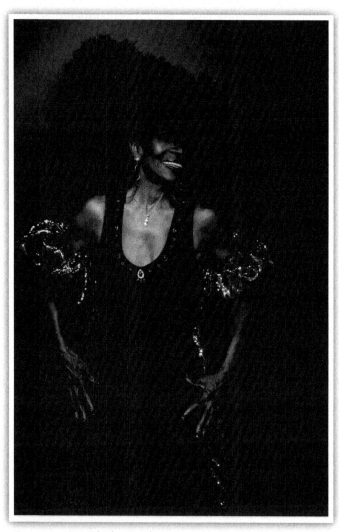

I am pictured above showcasing my modeling and acting abilities. The outfit I am wearing is what I wore to portray Josephine Baker at my church, Union Memorial United Methodist Church, during our Black History Month celebration on February 21, 2016.

Photo Credit: Marvin Joseph Photography